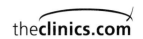
theclinics.com

CLINICS IN PODIATRIC MEDICINE AND SURGERY

The Charcot Foot

GUEST EDITOR
Lee C. Rogers, DPM

CONSULTING EDITOR
Vincent J. Mandracchia, DPM, MSHCA

January 2008 • Volume 25 • Number 1

SAUNDERS

An Imprint of Elsevier, Inc.
PHILADELPHIA   LONDON   TORONTO   MONTREAL   SYDNEY   TOKYO

W.B. SAUNDERS COMPANY
A Division of Elsevier Inc.

1600 John F. Kennedy Blvd., Suite 1800, Philadelphia, PA 19103-2899

http://www.theclinics.com

CLINICS IN PODIATRIC MEDICINE	Volume 25, Number 1
AND SURGERY	ISSN 0891-8422
January 2008	ISBN-13: 978-1-4160-5854-0
Editor: Patrick Manley	ISBN-10: 1-4160-5854-0

The ideas and opinion expressed in *Clinics in Podiatric Medicine and Surgery* do not necessarily reflect those of the Publisher. The Publisher does not assume any responsibility for any injury and/or damage to persons or property arising out of or related to any use of the material contained in this periodical. The reader is advised to check the appropriate medical literature and the product information currently provided by the manufacturer of each drug to be administered to verify the dosage, the method and duration of administration, or contraindications. It is the responsibility of the treating physician or other health care professional, relying on independent experience and knowledge of the patient, to determine drug dosages and the best treatment for the patient. Mention of any product in this issue should not be construed as endorsement by the contributors, editors, or the Publisher of the product of manufacturers' claims.

Reprints. For copies of 100 or more of articles in this publication, please contact the Commercial Reprints Department, Elsevier Inc., 360 Park Avenue South, New York, New York 10010-1710 Tel.: (212) 633-3813, Fax: (212) 462-1935, e-mail: reprints@elsevier.com

Clinics in Podiatric Medicine and Surgery (ISSN 0891-8422) is published quarterly by Elsevier Inc., 360 Park Avenue South, New York, NY 10010-1710. Months of publication are January, April, July, and October. Business and Editorial Offices: 1600 John F. Kennedy Blvd., Suite 1800, Philadelphia, PA 191023-2899. Customer Service Office: 6277 Sea Harbor Drive, Orlando, FL 32887-4800. Periodicals postage paid at New York, NY, and additional mailing offices. Subscription prices are $208.00 per year for US individuals, $327.00 per year for US institutions, $107.00 per year for US students and residents, $250.00 per year for Canadian individuals, $396.00 for Canadian institutions, $279.00 for international individuals, $396.00 per year for international institutions and $143.00 per year for Canadian and foreign students/residents. To receive student/resident rate, orders must be accompanied by name of affiliated institution, date of term, and the *signature* of program/residency coordinator on institution letterhead. Orders will be billed at individual rate until proof of status is received. Foreign air speed delivery is included in all *Clinics* subscription prices. All prices are subject to change without notice. POSTMASTER: Send address changes to *Clinics in Podiatric Medicine and Surgery*, Elsevier Periodicals Customer Service, 6277 Sea Harbor Drive, Orlando, FL 32887-4800. **Customer Service: 1-800-654-2452 (US). From outside of the US, call 1-407-345-1000.**

Clinics in Podiatric Medicine and Surgery is covered in *Index Medicus and EMBASE/Excerpta Medica.*

Printed in the United States of America.

CONSULTING EDITOR

VINCENT J. MANDRACCHIA, DPM, MSHCA, Chief Medical Officer; Staff Podiatrist, Section of Podiatric Surgery, Department of Surgery, Broadlawns Medical Center; Clinical Professor, Department of Podiatric Medicine and Surgery, College of Podiatric Medicine and Surgery, Des Moines University—Osteopathic Medicine Center, Des Moines, Iowa

GUEST EDITOR

LEE C. ROGERS, DPM, Director, Amputation Prevention Center, Broadlawns Medical Center, Des Moines, Iowa

CONTRIBUTORS

DAVID G. ARMSTRONG, DPM, PhD, Professor of Surgery and Associate Dean, Scholl's Center for Lower Extremity Ambulatory Research at Rosalind Franklin University of Medicine and Science, North Chicago, Illinois

TIMOTHY BARRY, DPM, AACFAS, Memorial Hospital and Healthcare Center, The Wound Care Center, Jasper, Indiana

RONALD BELCZYK, DPM, Resident, University of Pittsburgh Medical Center, Pittsburgh, Pennsylvania

NICHOLAS J. BEVILACQUA, DPM, Foot and Ankle Surgery, Amputation Prevention Center, Broadlawns Medical Center, Des Moines, Iowa

PATRICK R. BURNS, DPM, FACFAS, Clinical Assistant Professor of Orthopaedic Surgery, Foot and Ankle Division, University of Pittsburgh School of Medicine, Pittsburgh, Pennsylvania; and Residency Director, Podiatric Surgical Training Program, University of Pittsburgh Medical Center South Side Hospital, Pittsburgh, Pennsylvania

RYAN T. CREWS, MS, Clinical Research Scientist, Center for Lower Extremity Ambulatory Research (CLEAR), Instructor, Department of Biomechanics and Orthopedic Diseases, Dr. William M. Scholl College of Podiatric Medicine at Rosalind Franklin University of Medicine and Science, North Chicago, Illinois

MICHAEL P. DELLACORTE, DPM, Caritas Heathcare, Inc., Department of Podiatry, St. Johns Hospital, Elmhurst, New York

ROBERT G. FRYKBERG, DPM, MPH, Chief, Podiatry, Carl T Hayden Medical Center, Phoenix, Arizona

WILLIAM JEFFCOATE, MRCP, Professor, Consultant Endocrinologist, Foot Ulcer Trials Unit, Department of Diabetes and Endocrinology Nottingham University Hospitals Trust, City Hospital Campus, Nottingham, United Kingdom

ANDREAS JOSTEL, MD, Specialist Registrar, Tameside Acute NHS Trust, Ashton-under-Lyne, Lancashire, United Kingdom

EDWARD B. JUDE, MD, MRCP, Consultant Physician and Honorary Senior Lecturer, Tameside Acute NHS Trust, Ashton-under-Lyne, Lancashire, United Kingdom

DAVID L. NIELSON, DPM, Research Fellow, Center for Lower Extremity Ambulatory Research, Dr. William M. Scholl College of Podiatric Medicine at Rosalind Franklin University of Medicine and Science, North Chicago, Illinois

ANDREW RADER, DPM, FACFAOM, CWS, FAPWCA, Memorial Hospital and Healthcare Center, The Wound Care Center, Jasper, Indiana; St. Mary's Healthcare Center, The Diabetic Foot Clinic, Evansville, Indiana

LEE C. ROGERS, DPM, Director, Amputation Prevention Center, Broadlawns Medical Center, Des Moines, Iowa

LEE J. SANDERS, DPM, Chief, Podiatry Service, VA Medical Center, Lebanon, Pennsylvania; and Adjunct Clinical Professor Department of Podiatric Medicine, Temple University School of Podiatric Medicine, Philadelphia, Pennsylvania

JAMES S. WROBEL, DPM, MS, Associate Professor of Medicine, Director, Outcomes Research Program, Center for Lower Extremity Ambulatory Research (CLEAR), Dr. William M. Scholl College of Podiatric Medicine at Rosalind Franklin University of Medicine and Science, North Chicago, Illinois

DANE K. WUKICH, MD, Chief, Foot and Ankle Division and Assistant Professor of Orthopaedic Surgery University of Pittsburgh School of Medicine, Pittsburgh, Pennsylvania; Medical Director, University of Pittsburgh Medical Center, Comprehensive Foot and Ankle Center, Pittsburgh, Pennsylvania

CONTENTS

Regrettably, physicians today receive very little instruction in the history of medicine. Most health care providers have a very limited, contemporary knowledge of the condition that we know of as the Charcot foot. Yet, historical concepts of the pathogenesis and natural history of this condition provide us with important lessons that enhance our understanding, recognition, and management of this rare but debilitating neurogenic arthropathy. It is my belief that knowledge of the history of medicine provides us with a better understanding of present-day issues and clearer vision as we look to the future. This article describes some of the important lessons learned from the history of the Charcot foot.

The Charcot foot (osteoarthropathy) is a significant lower extremity complication of diabetes mellitus that can result in significant deformity, ulceration, and subsequent limb loss. A result of even unrecognized trauma to an insensitive foot, continued weight bearing on the injured foot promotes the evolution of the disorder that is often diagnosed only after significant deformity has occurred. Although this entity is considered a rare complication of the diabetic population, it has profound implications for those persons affected. Greater awareness of the frequency, distribution, determinants, and natural history of Charcot foot can help clinicians establish an earlier diagnosis and institute effective treatment before the onset of limb-threatening deformity.

pharmacological intervention are inhibition of excess osteoclast activation and suppression of an excess proinflammatory cytokine response. Antiresorptive therapy, especially with bisphosphonates, has been used in randomized trials. While evidence of an ideal dosage regime and significant differences in long-term outcome are lacking and should be evaluated in future studies, the trials so far demonstrated improved symptom control, a more rapid decline in foot temperature, and a significant decrease in bone turnover markers, with no demonstration of significant harmful effects. Growing insight into molecular pathways of resorptive bone disease will undoubtedly facilitate novel adjunctive pharmacological therapies.

Charcot arthropathy places individuals at risk of developing diabetic foot ulcers and potentially subsequent limb amputation by means of altering the anatomy of the foot and ankle. Physical trauma is an important component to the etiology of the condition. The physical management of the Charcot foot is concerned with minimizing the stress applied to the affected foot and ankle skeletal structure. The most appropriate device is temporally dependent on the progression of the disease. At the initiation of Charcot arthropathy, care by total contact cast is recommended. As the affected bones begin to heal, use of a removable cast walker may be implemented. When the bones reach a fixed state, appropriate footwear is dictated by the degree of deformity.

Diagnosing Charcot neuroarthropathy requires a heightened index of suspicion. Early recognition and intervention can limit deformity. Aggressive conservative management should be initiated early in the treatment plan to minimize the devastating effects often seen with this condition. Any delay in therapy can result in severe foot and ankle deformity in which traditional nonoperative methods alone may be inadequate. These deformities may lead to ulcerations and ultimately progress to amputation of the lower extremity. Surgical correction and stabilization is an effective method to prevent further deformity and ulcer recurrence. If performed in the appropriate setting and for the right indications, Charcot foot reconstruction is a better alternative to lower limb amputation.

Charcot arthropathy of the rearfoot and ankle is a complex disorder. To date there are no evidence-based, universally agreed upon treatment protocols. As the number of patients who have these deformities continues to increase, surgeons' skill levels and experience grow as well. With increased technical skill, knowledge, and advances in fixation, these deformities are becoming more manageable. In the future this experience should afford the general community with evidenced-based protocols. This article discusses basic techniques in deformity planning and current uses of internal and external fixation techniques for rearfoot and ankle limb salvage.

FORTHCOMING ISSUES

RECENT ISSUES

THE CLINICS ARE NOW AVAILABLE ONLINE!

http://www.theclinics.com

ELSEVIER
SAUNDERS

Clin Podiatr Med Surg
25 (2008) xi–xii

CLINICS IN
PODIATRIC
MEDICINE AND
SURGERY

Preface

The Charcot Foot

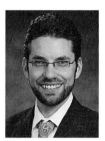

Lee C. Rogers, DPM
Guest Editor

"The good physician treats the disease; the great physician treats the patient who has the disease."

Sir William Osler, 1849–1919

The Charcot foot is a complex syndrome that frequently leads to disability, ulceration, and amputation. Its pathogenesis is becoming better understood, but frequently patients seek treatment too late or are unfortunately misdiagnosed at a time when interventions can interrupt the cycle of bone destruction and deformity.

This issue attempts to be a primer on Charcot foot and addresses the syndrome in an orderly and complete fashion. We have reviewed the literature to provide the reader with the most current recommendations on abortive medical treatments, accommodative physical therapies, and corrective surgical procedures. The section authors are researchers and recognized global authorities on their topics.

The issue is dedicated to those patients who suffer from this debilitating condition and to those who may have lost limbs unnecessarily. Extremity amputations are an unfortunate and sometimes avoidable cause of morbidity and mortality in this population. May we, physicians and surgeons, strive to increase our knowledge, clinical acumen, and compassion for those with Charcot foot.

0891-8422/08/$ - see front matter © 2008 Elsevier Inc. All rights reserved.
doi:10.1016/j.cpm.2007.11.001   *podiatric.theclinics.com*

I thank all the contributors for their hard work. I also thank my wife, Susan, for tolerating this worthwhile exercise during our cross-country move and recent wedding.

Lee C. Rogers, DPM
Director
Amputation Prevention Center
Broadlawns Medical Center
1801 Hickman Road
Des Moines, IA 50131, USA

E-mail address: Lee.C.Rogers@gmail.com

ELSEVIER
SAUNDERS

Clin Podiatr Med Surg
25 (2008) 1–15

CLINICS IN
PODIATRIC
MEDICINE AND
SURGERY

What Lessons Can History Teach Us About the Charcot Foot?

Lee J. Sanders, DPM[a,b,*]

[a]Podiatry Service (323), VA Medical Center, 1700 South Lincoln Avenue, Lebanon,
PA 17042, USA
[b]Department of Podiatric Medicine, Temple University School of Podiatric Medicine,
Philadelphia, PA, USA

Let us keep looking, in spite of everything. Let us keep searching. It is indeed the best method for finding, and perhaps, thanks to our efforts, the verdict we will give this patient tomorrow will not be the same as we must give him today [1].

J.-M. Charcot.

Regrettably, physicians today receive very little instruction in the history of medicine. Most health care providers have a very limited, contemporary knowledge of the condition that we know of as the Charcot foot. Yet, historical concepts of the pathogenesis and natural history of this condition provide us with important lessons that enhance our understanding, recognition and management of this rare but debilitating neurogenic arthropathy. It is my belief that knowledge of the history of medicine provides us with a better understanding of present-day issues and clearer vision as we look to the future. The following are some of the important lessons learned from the history of the Charcot foot.

Lesson number one: Observation is the clinical starting point

J.-M. Charcot (1825–1893) personified one of the greatest clinicians of the nineteenth century, one who knew how to see and to discover [2–5]. He was resolute in his belief that clinical observation was always the fundamental starting point, the first steps of every scientific theory in studying diseases. He taught that "theories no matter how pertinent they are, cannot eradicate the existence of facts" (Fig. 1) [3]. J.-M. Charcot transformed

---

* Corresponding author. Podiatry Service (323), VA Medical Center, 1700 South Lincoln Avenue, Lebanon, PA 17042.
  E-mail address: lee.sanders@med.va.gov

0891-8422/08/$ - see front matter. Published by Elsevier Inc.
doi:10.1016/j.cpm.2007.09.003

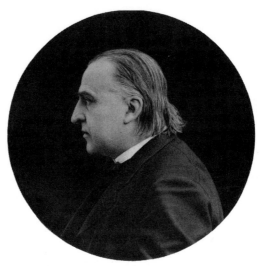

M. LE PROFESSEUR CHARCOT

DE L'ACADEMIE DES SCIENCES

Fig. 1. Jean-Martin Charcot. Charcot was appointed the first Clinical Professor (Chair) of Diseases of the Nervous System at the Paris Medical Faculty in 1882. He was elected to membership in the French Academy of Sciences on November 12, 1883. This represented the pinnacle of scientific recognition in France. Photoengraving by Albert Londe. Les Lettres Et Les Arts, L'Hypnotism. Revue Illustrée, Paris, 1886. (*From* the private collection of Dr Lee J. Sanders.)

the practice of medicine and neurologic research with his clinicoanatomic method (méthode anatomo-clinique). This two-part approach emphasized the importance of meticulous clinical observation, documentation, and classification as well as anatomic and histologic studies. Charcot was therefore able to correlate discrete lesions of the nervous system with various neurologic diseases. The clinicoanatomic method became the research discipline at the Salpêtrière, and enabled Charcot to transform this large charitable hospital in Paris, that he described as "a grand asylum of human misery...a museum of living pathology," [3] into a great teaching and research center for diseases of the nervous system (Fig. 2).

Charcot was the first to describe the arthropathies associated with tabes dorsalis (neurosyphilis), also known as progressive locomotor ataxia [1,6–9]. These two terms were used interchangeably to describe the same condition. The term "tabes dorsalis" was an anatomical description coined by Romberg, whereas "locomotor ataxia" was a clinical term selected by Duchenne de Boulogne. Charcot depicted the unique clinical manifestations of the tabetic arthropathies, as follows: *"There is a sudden onset of general tumefaction of the limb; rapid changes in the articular surfaces of the joint which manifest themselves as crepitations that are often noticed a few days after the onset, their appearance being evidently determined by the duration of the spinal cord disease..."* [3] He noted that the bone and joint changes preceded

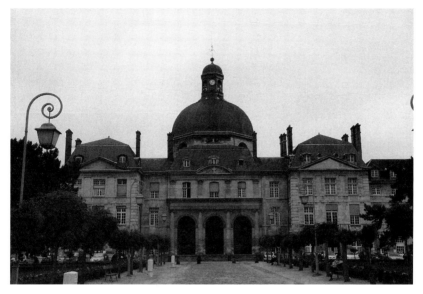

Fig. 2. Entrance to the Salpêtrière Hospital in Paris, as it appears today. During Charcot's tenure at the Salpêtrière, this was the largest charitable hospital in Europe. It was a women's asylum, described by Charcot as "a grand asylum of human misery...a museum of living pathology." The dome and central spire of the Saint-Louis Chapel are seen in the background.

the characteristic motor incoordination of locomotor ataxia. *"These arthropathies develop without apparent cause; they do not result exclusively, as has been claimed, from the distension undergone by the ligaments and capsules of the joints or from the awkward gaits characteristic of ataxic patients...Anatomically the enormous wear and tear shown by the heads of the bones, the extensive looseness of the ligaments of the joints, and the frequent occurrence of luxations seem to distinguish these arthropathies from the ordinary type of osteoarthritis"* [3]. Charcot concluded, *"...behind the disease of the joint was a disease far more important in character, and which in reality dominated the situation"* [8].

This assumption was correct; however, J.-M. Charcot failed to recognize the infectious etiology of tabes dorsalis as a long-term complication of tertiary syphilis; while asserting his belief that most neurologic disorders were hereditary. The definitive identification of tabes dorsalis as a form of tertiary syphilis would not occur until 1906 with the introduction of a serologic test for syphilis, the Wasserman test [1].

Charcot's attention to clinical histories revealed that patients with tabetic joints often experienced lightning-like pains, like a shower of electric needles, before the development of their arthropathies [1,6–9]. The pain was of short duration but recurrent throughout the day. At the same time, these pains were accompanied by loss of sensation and hyperesthesia. Charcot emphasized that, *"in diabetes you can have very similar complaints...you can also have absent deep tendon reflexes... Do not mistake a diabetic for a tabetic... there is still another disorder with lightening pains—alcoholic paralysis... the gait of the alcoholic can, in fact, resemble the patient with locomotor ataxia"* [1,9]. Charcot also noted that sensation to touch, pressure, and temperature in the lower extremities is decreased but not abolished [6,7].

Although J.-M. Charcot's early observations of the tabetic arthropathies were published in January 1868 [6], it was not until August 1881 that he received triumphant international acclaim for his research. Charcot presented his clinicoanatomic studies of patients with tabetic arthropathies at the 7th International Medical Congress, held in London in 1881. This meeting was described by *The Lancet* as *"a gathering the like of which has never been witnessed before, and in all probability will never be paralleled in our day"* [5]. Charcot's presentation was entitled, "Demonstration of Arthropathic Affections of Locomotor Ataxy" [10,11]. He demonstrated his presentation with the wax model of a 60-year old woman, named Berthelot, showing the character of ataxic affections of the joints. The wax model was accompanied by the complete skeleton of the patient, and by serial photographs taken at different stages of the disease. In addition, Charcot presented a variety of characteristic anatomical specimens of bones and joints, and sections of the spine demonstrating posterior sclerosis of the spinal cord. He remarked, *"when the disease attacks the diaphyses of the bone, the atrophy is shown by fracture; when it attacks the joint we get wasting of the head of the bone, with an erosion of the surface"* [10,11]. In the Transactions of the International Medical Congress, it was recorded that *"This disease is, in fact, a distinct pathological entity, and deserves the name, by which it will be known, of 'Charcot's disease' "* [10]. The eponyms, "Charcot's joint disease" and "Charcot's arthropathy," have since been adopted in reference to all neuropathic arthropathies, regardless of their etiology.

It is interesting to note that Charcot's demonstration at the 7th International Medical Congress did not mention bone and joint involvement of the foot or ankle. However, at this same meeting, a lesser-known English physician, Herbert W. Page, presented a unique case of a 30-year-old man with bilateral joint disease of the foot and ankle in a case of tabes dorsalis [10]. Without hesitancy Page associated the bone and joint changes that he observed in this patient, with the group of tabetic arthropathies. *"Of the rarity of this particular form of arthropathy there can be little doubt, and Charcot himself remarked when he saw the case in London that only one instance of the same kind had fallen under his observation"* [12].

Lesson number two: Suspicion of the Charcot foot and early recognition are of utmost importance

Herbert W. Page noted the practical importance of recognizing this rare condition, and believed that the duty for this rested with the generalist physician. *"It is by the surgeons of general hospitals, not by physicians of special hospitals, that these cases must be recognized and recorded...And the practical importance of this recognition is abundantly shown by the history of this case. Had his left foot been the first affection seen, as it was seen on July 21, 1881, there can be little doubt that the foot would have been at once condemned and forthwith removed. It was by a mere accident, as it were, in the development of his symptoms that the patient still has his foot, deformed it is true, but better than any artificial limb"* [12].

In the case presented by Herbert W. Page, his suspicion was aroused by the absolute painlessness of the very angry looking ulcers on the sole of his patient's foot. This finding led him to closer examination. He noted that the deep tendon reflexes were absent at the knee in both limbs and the patient was unsteady on his feet when standing with his eyes shut. *"When shown at the Congress on August 6, the swelling of the right foot had much subsided, and the bones, originally involved, seemed anchylosed* (sic) *together. The left foot, however, had gone on from bad to worse. It had gradually increased in size...the ankle suddenly slipping on one side. Crepitus could be obtained at the ankle joint, and the foot gave the sensation on handling of being a mere bag of loose bones. Manipulation was painless. Such a foot would, indeed, have called for immediate removal had not the nature of this case been known, and had not the subsidence of the swelling and the anchylosis* (sic) *of the bones of his right foot suggested the advisability of leaving his left foot alone. It was therefore secured in a plaster-of-Paris bandage"* [12].

Herbert W. Page recorded what may be the earliest description of a *rocker-bottom* foot deformity, associated with a tabetic arthropathy. He observed, *"The sole of this foot is $4\frac{3}{4}$ inches wide, and there runs across it, midway between the heel and the toes, a hard transverse ridge, composed doubtless of the tarsal bones, for the base of the first metatarsal bone has no longer a cuneiform bone to articulate with, and stands out as an abrupt projection on the dorsum. On this transverse ridge his foot rests on the ground, and you are able to get the tip of your little finger underneath his heel when he is standing"* [12]. This *rocker-bottom* deformity has become the hallmark of midfoot collapse in the Charcot foot.

Prior to 1883, nearly all published observations of bone and joint lesions of the ataxic were of the long bones of the limbs and their large articulations. However, in April 1883, Herbert W. Page read the history of his case to the Clinical Society of London. This was the very same case that was originally shown by him in 1881 at the International Medical Congress. In November 1883, Charcot and Féré published their first observations of the bone and joint conditions of the tabetic foot (pied tabétique), in the *Archives de Neurologie* [13]. My translation of the introduction to this paper begins, *"Described for the first time, by one of us, the bone and joint conditions of the ataxic are well recognized today, at least their general features, when located on the long bones of the limbs and their large joints... Similar changes corresponding to the short bones and small joints of the foot have not yet been the subject of published observations. It is these findings that we wish to call attention to."* Charcot and Féré presented five observations of tabetic patients with locomotor ataxia, lancinating pains, and foot deformities. This paper marks the first published case series and scientific investigation of tabetic arthropathy of the foot, *pied tabétique.* One of these observations, *Observation II,* was the case presented by Herbert W. Page, at the International Medical Congress, on August 6, 1881.

The following is an excerpt from the first case observed by Charcot and Féré.

It was in the month of April 1881, that they observed the first example of this condition.

"Observation I—Locomotor Ataxia. Laryngeal crises. Disorders of micturition. Lancinating pain, anesthesia, incoordination, oculo-pupillary phenomenon. Deformity of the feet."

The patient is a 41-year-old male who presented in consultation to the Salpêtrière on April 30, 1881. In January 1879 he began to experience lancinating pains in his legs. In the month of September 1879 he began to suffer deformity of his feet. At that time, he believed he had a sprain; but he had no memory of a traumatic injury. The affected parts were a little painful, but not enough to prevent him from walking. Loss of sensation was nearly complete in his feet and legs, with motor incoordination and positive Romberg's sign. Reflexes were absent in his both legs. The two feet had exactly the same deformity, but more pronounced on the right. The medial border of the foot was considerably increased in thickness in all the parts that corresponded to the navicular, first cuneiform and the tarso-metatarsal articulation. In addition, the metatarsals were deviated to the outside. At the level of the tarso-metatarsal articulation there was a strongly projecting angle. Cracking sounds (crepitations) were not observed at the level of the deformed parts (Fig. 3).

Charcot and Féré believed that, in the absence of anatomic verification in this first case, they should reserve their opinion relative to the intimate nature of this condition. They sufficiently believed that this was a tabetic arthropathy and provisionally designated their findings by the name *pied tabétique,* until proven by other observations and investigations [13].

In a fifth observation, Charcot and Féré discuss the gross examination of a skeleton foot in a complex case with extensive bone and joint destruction (Fig. 4). They concluded their discussion by stating that the complex condition of the small bones and joints of the foot is analogous to the tabetic arthropathies affecting the long bones and large joints, which develop in the course of locomotor ataxia. For the sake of convenience they proposed the designation of the term *pied tabétique.* This condition would come to be known as the Charcot foot.

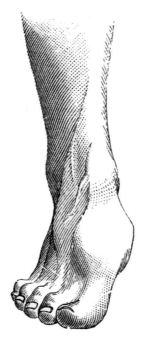

Fig. 3. Arthropathy of the right foot. Observation I, the first case of *pied tabétique* observed by J.-M. Charcot and Charles Féré at the Salpêtrière, April 30, 1881. (*From* Charcot J-M, Féré C. Affections osseuses et articulaires du pied chez les tabétiques [Pied tabétique]: *Archives de Neurologie* 1883;6(18):305–19. *Courtesy of* the New York Academy of Medicine, New York, NY.)

Lesson number three: Gait analysis and foot structure have important diagnostic significance

Charcot organized a gait laboratory where he and his students studied the gait of their patients. He recognized that a patient's gait had important diagnostic significance for certain diseases, and he taught his students to listen to patient's walking patterns [1]. Specifically, he trained them to listen for the contact of the foot with the ground. Joseph Babinski wrote, in his Preface to the Leçons Mardi (Tuesday Lessons), *"In one case, a single glance at the patient, his movement, his speech or his gait will suffice to give the case away"* [1,9]. Charcot compared the gait of a patient with alcoholic polyneuropathy (with foot drop), to one with tabes, as follows: "*If the ankle flexors and extensors are affected, as is sometimes the case, the foot will be absolutely flaccid. As the patient walks, he over flexes at the knee joint and the thigh lifts upward more than it should. As the foot hits the ground, the toes hit first and then the heel, so that you can quite distinctively hear two successive sounds. In this example, the alcoholic bends his knees excessively like a prancing horse, resulting in a steppage gait. However, the ataxic patient thrusts his legs forward in extension with almost no flexion at the knee joint; this time the foot hits the ground all at once, making only a single noise*" (Fig. 5) [1,9].

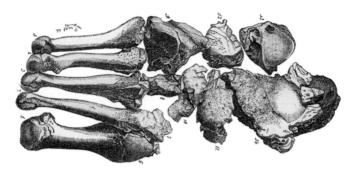

Fig. 4. Skeleton of the ataxic foot, a complex case: 1, 2, 3, 4, 5, metatarsals; 6, 7, first and second cuneiforms fused to their corresponding metatarsals; 8, bony fragment apparently the third cuneiform; 9, the cuboid is represented by an irregular mass and can be recognized only by the (peroneal) groove on the inferior surface; 10, 11, two fragments of the navicular; 12, 13, neck and body of the talus. The talar head has disappeared, and the superior surface of the body is completely worn down; 14, the calcaneus. The articular surface of the posterior facet is easily recognizable. There are a number of small osteophytes noted. The anterior facet is completely worn down. (*From* Charcot J-M, Féré C. Affections osseuses et articulaires du pied chez les tabétiques [Pied tabétique]: *Archives de Neurologie* 1883;6(18):305–19. *Courtesy of* the New York Academy of Medicine, New York, NY.)

Additional diagnostic information on foot structure was collected using inked footprints. This provided both qualitative and quantitative data on foot shape, stride length, and width [1,5].

Footprints were used to distinguish between foot deformities associated with various neurologic disorders. *"With tabes, the foot deformity relates to an erosion of the tarsal bones, with a resultant flat foot, and especially marked protrusions of the medial tarsal components. In such cases, the flat foot seems enlarged, and a footprint would show an impression for the entire foot"* [1].

Lesson number four: Diabetes is the leading cause of the Charcot foot today

The association between Charcot's joint disease of the foot and ankle and diabetes mellitus was established for the first time in 1936, by William Riely Jordan [14]. Since this early report by Jordan, the number of case reports of the diabetic Charcot foot has steadily increased. As the number of cases of tabes dorsalis (neurosyphylis) has declined, diabetes has emerged as the leading cause of neurogenic arthropathy today [15]. The increased prevalence of the diabetic form of neuropathic arthropathy was established in 1955 in a report by Miller and Lichtman at the Cook County Hospital and Chicago Medical School [16]. They noted that *"whereas tabes of syphilitic origin was formerly the usual cause of these painless deformities of the feet, with complicating soft tissue infections, ulcers and osteomyelitis, the diabetic neuropathic foot is now showing the higher incidence"* [16]. Some classic observations of the emerging diabetic Charcot foot, published in the twentieth century, will follow in the next lesson on treatment for this condition.

PUBLICATIONS DU *PROGRÈS MÉDICAL*

LEÇONS DU MARDI A LA SALPÊTRIÈRE

Professeur CHARCOT

POLICLINIQUE

1887-1888

Notes de Cours de MM. BLIN, CHARCOT, Henri COLIN,

ÉLÈVES DU SERVICE

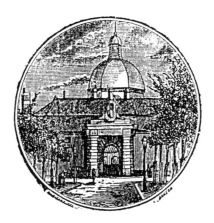

PARIS

AUX BUREAUX DU
PROGRÈS MÉDICAL
14, rue des Carmes. 14.

E. LECROSNIER & BABÉ
ÉDITEURS
Place de l'École de Médecine

1888

Fig. 5. Front piece, *Leçons du Mardi à la Salpêtrière*, Polycliniques 1887–1888, Notes de Cours de MM. Blin, Charcot, Henri Colin. Bureaux du Progrès Médical, Paris. 1888. The Tuesday Lessons emphasized everyday general neurology. These were teaching sessions designed to teach doctors how to treat patients with neurological diseases. The lessons were recorded by J.-M. Charcot's students. (*Courtesy of* the National Library of Medicine, Bethesda, MD.)

Lesson number five: Treatment of the Charcot foot is prolonged and challenging

Nonpharmacologic therapies for treatment of the tabetic arthropathies, during the nineteenth century, consisted of bed rest, firm bandage support, hydrotherapy, electrotherapies, physical rehabilitation, and off-loading of the foot. Herbert W. Page used a plaster-of-Paris bandage. One of the most extraordinary therapies employed by Charcot for the treatment of locomotor ataxia and other neurological diseases was suspension therapy (Fig. 6). Most patients treated with suspension therapy were tabetics. This treatment was introduced by Charcot, at a Polyclinique Tuesday Lesson, on January 15, 1889 [9]. The concept for this therapy was nerve stretching, for the relief or cure of lancinating pain. A suspension apparatus was applied to the patient's head and chin, and then a therapist hoisted the patient into the air. Patients were suspended for a maximum of 4 minutes at each session. The treatment was very painful and posed a physical risk to the subject. In one case, a patient with multiple sclerosis became suddenly paraplegic after two sessions [5]. This therapy was soon abandoned by Charcot. I have used the illustration of this therapy in my lectures on the Charcot foot to introduce the concept of off-loading. Suspension therapy was the quintessential approach to removing weight-bearing stress from the lower limbs. As you will see, investigators continue to search for a safe and effective method to off-load, protect, and stabilize the neuropathic foot.

In the twentieth century we begin to see scattered reports of neuropathic arthropathies affecting the feet. At first these reports were focused on patients with neurosyphilis; however, we soon witness a shift of attention to patients with diabetes mellitus and leprosy. Arthur Steindler, in his 1931 discussion of the treatment of the tabetic arthropathies, noted the importance of immediate and adequate protection of the joint to prevent detrimental external influences. He advised early and adequate splinting, preservation of protecting musculature by physical therapy, "*and above all, earliest stabilization and alignment by conservative or operative means* [17]."

In 1947, Bailey and Root reported on a series of 17 neuropathic foot lesions (bone and joint destruction) in patients with diabetes [18]. Bone destruction was chiefly limited to the tarsal bones and proximal ends of the metatarsal bones. The authors concluded that the bone destruction in these patients represented trophic changes resulting from diabetic neuropathy, similar to the arthropathies seen from neurosyphilis and leprosy. None of the cases showed any tendency to get better, and in most cases destruction gradually progressed. *"No treatment proved efficacious, but orthopedic appliances were used in an effort to relieve weight-bearing and to avoid further deformity."*

In 1955, Miller and Lichtman presented another small series of 17 diabetic patients with neuropathic arthropathy of their feet [16]. They wrote that *"diabetic neuropathic arthropathies of the feet are grave, often leading*

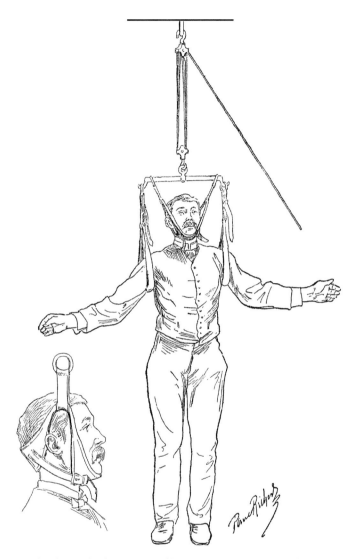

Fig. 6. Suspension therapy for the treatment of locomotor ataxia. Illustration by Paul Richer in Polyclinique du Mardi 15 Janvier 1889. Dixième Leçon. *Leçons du Mardi à la Salpêtrière*, Polycliniques 1888–1889. Pages 206 and 208. (*Courtesy of* the National Library of Medicine, Bethesda, MD.)

to total disability, with reduction or even loss of gainful occupation. Treatment is empirical and conservative, and the prognosis must be guarded.'' They remarked that surgical intervention with ostectomy or fusion, was indicated only when deformity was severe and weight bearing difficult.

In 1966, Harris and Brand published a classic paper on tarsal disintegration in leprosy [19]. They drew attention to the importance of immobilization and off-loading the foot, as well as successful surgical fusion: *''short of complete rest in bed nothing less than immobilization in a plaster boot is adequate...If it is not possible to restore pain sensibility to the foot it is at least possible to limit vigorous activity... In cases where joints are disintegrating, prolonged immobilization may still produce arrest of the process, but failure is common and surgical fusion should not be delayed if conservative methods are not successful. Charcot's joints have a bad reputation for non-union after surgical fusion, but we have success 1) if the operation is done early, and 2) in late cases so long as: the joints are excised boldly back to normal-looking bone...."*

The orthopedic surgeon J.T.H. Johnson echoed the importance of preventive therapy [20]. He noted that the prevailing attitude toward treatment of neuropathic fractures and joint injuries in the orthopedic literature was often rather pessimistic, normally recommending only bracing or arthrodesis. He advised that *"if we substitute protection for further trauma the result will be a healed fracture instead of a disorganized joint. However the protection must be adequate and sufficiently prolonged."* Johnson advocated that the proper way to treat Charcot joints is first to prevent them by warning neuropathic patients to protect themselves from trauma and their joints from overuse. His second major point in treatment was early recognition. *"It is vitally important to be on the lookout for any areas of mild swelling, local heat, and early instability or deformity."* He cautioned that postoperative infection is a great hazard after surgery on any neuropathic joint. *"The part should be kept at rest and surgery in most cases should be postponed until the area is no longer abnormally warm to the touch, and roentgenograms indicate repair rather than resorption. Neuropathic foot deformities are best treated by protection from weight-bearing until the acute process subsides and then by correcting deformities by such procedures as triple arthrodesis and the excision of any bony prominences that interfere with weight-bearing or the wearing of a shoe"* [20].

In 1972, Sinha and colleagues [21] reported on a large clinical study of 101 cases of Charcot joints in patients with diabetes mellitus. This comprehensive survey of patients seen at the New England Deaconess Hospital, confirmed the benefit of no weight bearing. They advised that the duration of treatment be determined according to clinical and radiological response. The role of surgery was less well defined. *"Only one of our patients was subjected to arthrodesis and results were equivocal. Clearly, there is a need for evaluation of this form of treatment in a substantial number of patients with stable disease...to minimize or avoid complications."*

History has taught us that the starting point for treatment of the diabetic Charcot foot is early recognition, followed by prolonged immobilization and off-loading of the foot until inflammation has subsided and the foot is stable. We have learned that therapeutic footwear and bracing are integral components of the approach to treatment. Patient education is an essential tool. High-risk individuals must be educated to understand the implications of sensory loss, as well as the importance of diabetes self-management.

Surgery should be contemplated when attempts at conservative care have failed to establish a stable, plantigrade foot or to prevent plantar ulceration. Advances in surgical techniques have resulted in better surgical outcomes, however complication rates are still high [15]. Long-term surgical outcome studies are needed to assess function and quality of life.

Lesson number six: Long-term surgical outcomes including functional evaluations and quality-of-life studies comparing alternative methods of treatment are lacking

Although external skeletal fixation is an accepted surgical approach for the correction of chronic severe foot and ankle deformities, the application of frames is still controversial with respect to the surgical management of the diabetic Charcot foot. Treatment is lengthy, frames are cumbersome, and complication rates are high. This is especially problematic for a uniquely vulnerable population of patients with diabetes and multiple co-morbidities. The threat of complications is significant for these patients, many who have cardiovascular risk factors, peripheral neuropathy, nutritional deficiency, and who may also be immunocompromised. There is a paucity of literature on the use of external fixation in the treatment of the Charcot foot. Most published studies are small, anecdotal, short-term, and retrospective. Long-term outcomes including functional evaluations and quality-of-life studies comparing alternative methods of treatment are needed.

Lesson number seven: Nomenclature for the Charcot foot is confusing

There is a lack of consensus on the nomenclature for noninfective bone disease in the neuropathic foot [15,22]. Newman described six different conditions of noninfective bone and joint pathology in patients with diabetic neuropathy, "Charcot osteoarthropathy" and "bone loss" were the most common conditions seen [23]. Uniform terminology needs to be adopted so as to avoid confusion over the diagnosis and treatment of this condition. With deference to J.-M. Charcot, my preferences are the following eponyms: Charcot's joint disease, the Charcot foot, and Charcot's osteoarthropathy. The latter term is most appropriate in that it refers to disease of bones (osteo) and joints (arthropathy).

Numerous other names and their variations have been used to describe neuropathic bone and joint disease. Some of these names include Charcot's disease, Charcot's joint, Charcot's arthropathy, Charcot neuroarthropathy, Charcot osteoarthropathy, Charcot neuropathic osteoarthropathy, diabetic osteopathy, diabetic neuropathic osteoarthropathy, diabetic osteoarthropathy, diabetic neuropathic arthropathy, diabetic neuroarthropathy, and neurogenic arthropathy.

The final lesson

In the first decade of the twenty-first century, we still have an incomplete understanding of the pathogenesis and treatment of the diabetic Charcot foot. Recognition of this condition, especially in its earliest stage remains problematic, with many cases going undiagnosed or misdiagnosed. Medical management remains the standard of care for most cases. Sadly, we have yet to find a way to prevent the occurrence of this condition. So, after 125 years of investigation, since Charcot and Féré's 1883 publication, it is still necessary to submit this condition to the control of new observations and research. It bears remembering the words of J.-M. Charcot: *"Let us keep looking, in spite of everything. Let us keep searching. It is indeed the best method for finding, and perhaps, thanks to our efforts, the verdict we will give this patient tomorrow will not be the same as we must give him today"* [1].

Acknowledgments

I acknowledge the assistance of Miriam Mandelbaum, Curator, and Arlene Shaner, Assistant Curator and reference librarian, Historical Collections, The New York Academy of Medicine.

References

[1] Charcot J-M. Charcot, the clinician: The Tuesday lessons: excerpts from nine case presentations on general neurology delivered at the Salpêtrière Hospital in 1887–88, trans by CG Goetz. New York: Raven Press; 1987.

[2] Cornil V. Banquet offert à M. le Prof. Charcot. Archives de Neurologie 1892;29:444–51 [in French].

[3] Guillain G. J.-M. Charcot 1825–1893: his life-his work [edited and translated by Pearce Bailey]. New York: Paul B. Hoeber; 1959.

[4] Sanders LJ. Jean-Martin Charcot (1825–1893). The man behind the joint disease. J Am Podiatr Med Assoc 2002;92(7):375–80.

[5] Goetz CG, Bonduelle M, Gelfand T. Charcot constructing neurology. New York: Oxford University Press; 1995.

[6] Charcot J-M. Sur quelques arthropathies qui paraissent dépendre d'une lésion du cerveau ou de la moelle épinière. Arch Physio Norm Pathol 1868;1:161–78 [in French].

[7] Hoché G, Sanders LJ. On some arthropathies apparently related to a lesion of the brain or spinal cord, by Dr. J.-M. Charcot, January 1868. J Hist Neurosci 1992;1(1):75–87.

[8] Charcot J-M. Lecture IV, on some visceral derangements in locomotor ataxia. Arthropathies of ataxic patients. In Lectures on the diseases of the nervous system, translated and edited by G. Sigerson. New York: Hafner; 1962.

[9] Charcot JM. Leçons du Mardi à la Salpêtrière, Polycliniques 1887–1888, 1888–1889, Notes de Cours de MM. Blin, Charcot, Henri Colin. Bureaux du Progrès Médical, Paris; 1888 [in French].

[10] MacCormac W, Klockmann JW. Transactions of the international medical congress: seventh session held in London, August 2–9, 1881. Vol 1. London: Balantyne, Hanson & Co.; 1881.

[11] Charcot J-M. Demonstration of arthropathic affections of locomotor ataxy. BMJ 1881;2: 285.

[12] Page HW. A case of tabetic arthropathy in which the tarsal bones of both feet were involved. By Herbert W. Page, M.C., F.R.C.S. Read April 13, 1883. Transactions of the Clinical Society of London 1882–1883;16:158–63.

[13] Charcot J-M, Féré C. Affections osseuses et articulaires du pied chez les tabétiques (Pied tabétique). Archives de Neurologie 1883;6(18):305–19 [in French].

[14] Jordan WR. Neuritic manifestations in diabetes mellitus. Arch Intern Med 1936;57:307–66.

[15] Sanders LJ, Frykberg RG. The Charcot foot (Pied de Charcot). In: John H, Bowker, Michael A, Pfeifer, editors. Levin and O'Neal's the diabetic foot. 7th edition. Philadelphia: Elsevier; 2007.

[16] Miller DS, Lichtman WF. Diabetic neuropathic arthropathy of feet: summary report of seventeen cases. AMA Arch Surg 1955;70(4):513–8.

[17] Steindler A. The tabetic arthropathies. JAMA 1931;96:250–6.

[18] Bailey CC, Root HF. Neuropathic foot lesions in diabetes mellitus. N Engl J Med 1947; 236(11):397–401.

[19] Harris JR, Brand PW. Patterns of disintegration of the tarsus in the anaesthetic foot. J Bone Joint Surg Br 1966;48(1):4–16.

[20] Johnson JT. Neuropathic fractures and joint injuries. Pathogenesis and rationale of prevention and treatment. J Bone Joint Surg Am 1967;49(1):1–30.

[21] Sinha S, Munichoodappa CS, Kozak GP. Neuro-arthropathy (Charcot joints) in diabetes mellitus (clinical study of 101 cases). Medicine (Baltimore) 1972;51(3):191–210.

[22] Foster AV. Problems with the nomenclature of Charcot's osteoarthropathy. The Diabetic Foot Journal 2005;8(3).

[23] Newman JH. Non-infective disease of the diabetic foot. J Bone Joint Surg Br 1981;63B(4): 593–6.

ELSEVIER
SAUNDERS

Clin Podiatr Med Surg
25 (2008) 17–28

CLINICS IN
PODIATRIC
MEDICINE AND
SURGERY

Epidemiology of the Charcot Foot

Robert G. Frykberg, DPM, MPH[a],*,
Ronald Belczyk, DPM[b]

[a]Carl T. Hayden Medical Center, 650 E. Indian School Road, Phoenix, AZ 85012, USA
[b]University of Pittsburgh Medical Center - South Side, 2000 Mary Street,
Pittsburgh, PA 15203, USA

The roots of epidemiology first originated with Hippocrates (460–377 BC). His classic work "On Airs, Waters, and Places" discussed the link between the environment and human health. He is known as the "father of modern epidemiology," since his contributions were the first documented use of observational techniques that led to accurate descriptions of diseases such as tetanus and malaria [1].

Today, epidemiology continues to use observational techniques to study the distribution and determinants of health-related states or events, populations, and the application of knowledge obtained to control health problems [2]. There are many areas of epidemiology. Of particular interest is the epidemiology of diabetes and the Charcot foot. There are various measurements typically used in epidemiology including occurrence, distribution, risk factors, morbidity, and mortality, all of which help determine clinical guidelines for managing neuropathic osteoarthopathy.

Charcot osteoarthropathy is an extremely destructive joint disorder affecting single or multiple joints that is almost uniformly initiated by trauma to an insensate limb or region. Those individuals acutely affected exhibit typical signs of inflammation (edema, erythema, and warmth) but generally without the protective sensation of pain. Fracture, dislocation, and instability of multiple joints within the foot or ankle are commonly seen [3,4]. The process can potentially result in collapse of the foot and severe deformity that frequently results in gait abnormalities and ulcer formation [5,6]. Characteristically, the entire process leading to gross deformities of the foot and/or ankle is relatively painless [7,8].

---

* Corresponding author.
E-mail address: robert.frykberg@va.gov (R.G. Frykberg).

0891-8422/08/$ - see front matter © 2008 Elsevier Inc. All rights reserved.
doi:10.1016/j.cpm.2007.10.001
podiatric.theclinics.com

Musgrave, in 1703, first reported neuropathic joint changes as a complication of venereal disease [9]. Then in 1831 Mitchell noted a connection between rheumatism and peripheral joint disorders [10]. In 1868, Jean Martin Charcot, perhaps one of the most famous physicians of his time, provided detailed descriptions of neuropathic osteoarthropathy in patients with tabes dorsalis [9,10]. However, only after his presentation, *Demonstration of Arthropathic Affections of Locomotor Ataxy*, at the 7th International Medical Congress (1881), did "pied tabetique" become established as a distinct pathological entity [11]. By 1936, Jordon associated neuropathic osteoarthropathy as a neuropathic complication in patients with diabetes [9–11]. While complications of tabes dorsalis have decreased, those of diabetes mellitus have increased. In more recent times diabetes has become the most common etiology for the development of neuropathic osteoarthropathy [9]. Hence, the term Diabetic Neuropathic Osteoarthropathy (DNOAP) has been used to describe such changes in the feet and ankles of patients with diabetes [5].

Disorders producing Charcot joints

Aside from diabetes mellitus and tabes dorsalis, there are a variety of other disorders with neuropathic manifestations in which Charcot joints can develop (Box 1). An exposure to toxic agents, infection (ie, syphilis,

---

Box 1. Disorders that have the potential to produce Charcot joints

Amyloidosis
Alcoholism
Cerebral palsy
Charcot Marie tooth
Congenital insensitivity to pain
Diabetes
Idiopathic sensorimotor neuropathy
Infection
Leprosy
Pernicious anemia
Poliomyelitis
Steroids
Syphilis
Surgery
Syringomyelia
Spina bifida
Spinal or peripheral nerve injury
Trauma

---

leprosy), and spinal and/or peripheral nerve injury have been known to cause this destructive pathology.

A chronic exposure to toxic agents like alcohol and corticosteroids are reported as potential risk factors for Charcot arthropathy.It is thought that the analgesic effect of steroids leads to overuse of a previously damaged joint, which results in accelerated cartilage deterioration [12]. Neuroarthropathy associated with infection such as tabes dorsalis or leprosy is more common in developing nations. Tabes dorsalis is a type of neurosyphilis in which the posterior roots of the spinal cord are involved and is seen in 10% to 20% of patients [13]. Leprosy, also known as Hansen's disease, is a chronic granulomatous infection caused by *Mycobacterium leprae* [2,14]. It most commonly affects the tibial nerve. Between 3% and 5% of hospitalized patients with leprosy have osseous changes in the small bones of the face, hands, and feet. Syringomyelia is caused by presence of longitudinal cavities lined by dense, gliogenous tissue in the spinal cord; Charcot arthropathy can been seen in 15% to 20% of patients [13]. The common feature of these disorders is the loss or decrease in pain sensation subsequent to nerve injury, disease, or metabolic dysfunction. With continued weight bearing, the initial bone stress injury or joint sprain worsens, eventually developing into an acute Charcot deformity [8].

Incidence, prevalence, and patient characteristics

Several population-based studies report an incidence of DNOAP in the range of 0.10% to −29.00%, whereas the prevalence varies between 0.08% and 13.00% (Tables 1 and 2) [3,5,15–19]. These studies also indicate a general trend for higher frequency in patients with peripheral neuropathy and those who present in specialty clinics [9]. Although the exact prevalence of Charcot

Table 1
Incidence of diabetic neuropathic osteoarthropathy

Reference	No. cases (np. feet or ankles)	Incidence
Sinha et al (1971)	101 (NA)	0.1%
Cofield et al (1983)	96 (116)	7.5% to 29.0%
Sella et al (1999)	40 (51)	5%
Fabrin and Holstein (2000)	115 (140)	0.3%/y
Sanders et al (2001)	N/A	0.1% to 7.5%
Rajbhandari (2002)	N/A	0.1% to 0.4%
Hartemann-Heurtier et al (2002)	N/A	0.2% to 3%
Lavery et al (2003)	N/A	Total: 8.5/1000/y Whites: 11.7/1000 Mexican American: 6.4/1000

Abbreviation: N/A, not available.

Table 2
Prevalence of diabetic neuropathic osteoarthropathy

Reference	Prevalence
Sanders et al (2001)	0.08% to 7.5%
Armstong et al (2001)	0.16% to 13.00%
Rajbhandari (2002)	0.1% to 0.4%

deformity is unknown, Sinha and colleagues found that 1 (0.15%) in 680 patients with diabetes developed osteoarthropathy in a large specialty referral center [17]. Armstrong later reported a prevalence of approximately 0.16% in a general population of patients with diabetes and a 13% prevalence in high-risk diabetic patients presenting to a foot clinic [9]. While the disorder affects about 0.2% of diabetic patients, minor joint changes can be noted in up to 3.0% [17]. However, in diabetic patients with established peripheral neuropathy, Cofield found a prevalence of radiographic changes in 29% of 333 patients [15,20].

The actual incidence of Charcot osteoarthropathy is perhaps greater than that reported because of diagnostic delays [11]. The diagnosis is delayed or missed in as many as 25% of patients [21,22] because the Charcot foot is not widely recognized by nonspecialists. The failure to identify the condition in its early phases is in part responsible for gross deformity that follows continued weight bearing [10,23].

Of the 24 patients Chantelau reviewed, 11 patients were referred early and 13 had delayed referrals. Based on the radiographs, 19 of 24 were misdiagnosed before referral. With the delayed referrals, 12 of 13 patients developed severe deformity. When referred early and immediate off-loading instituted, only 1 of 11 patients developed a severe deformity [23]. In a retrospective review of 36 cases, Pakarinen and colleagues [24] reported a diagnostic delay of an average of 29 weeks, while another retrospective review reported a delay in proper diagnosis of up to 6 months [25].

Often presenting initially with erythema, edema, and warmth, patients with early Charcot changes are frequently mismanaged as having cellulitis, venous thrombosis, gout, or sprains [25]. Often, requests are made from a surgeon to perform a bone biopsy to rule out an underlying source of osteomyelitis. When the early signs of the disease process are not recognized, proper off-loading with immobilization is not instituted and structural deformity occurs. The possibility of a Charcot process should therefore be among the differential diagnoses when examining a neuropathic diabetic patient with a swollen foot [4,8,23].

As documented by several studies, diabetes is now the primary cause of Charcot neuroarthropathy [18], but few studies have investigated an association with race or ethnicity. Lavery and colleagues [26] evaluated the prevalence and incidence of foot pathology in 1666 Mexican Americans and non-Hispanic whites enrolled in a disease management program for a period of 24 months. The incidence of Charcot arthropathy was 8.5/1000 per year.

They also found that Charcot deformities were more common in non-Hispanic whites than Mexican Americans, 11.7/1000 versus 6.4/1000, respectively. Additional research is needed to identify the variables for ethnic differences in the incidence of Charcot arthropathy. Moreover, it is important to appreciate perspectives of Charcot foot from other parts of the world.

McIntyre and colleagues [27] retrospectively reviewed clinical histories of Canadian aboriginal and nonaboriginal diabetic populations with end-stage renal disease. Their findings suggest that there are a significantly greater number of lower extremity complications in the aboriginal patients, including the number of Charcot presentations. The aboriginal diabetic population presented with a 23% frequency of a Charcot, while it was 17% respectively in the nonaboriginal population.The aboriginal population also had a significantly greater frequency of other lower extremity complications including ulcers, osteomyelitis, and amputations.

As the medical treatment of diabetes improves and patients live longer, it is likely that foot and ankle specialists will see more complications as a result of neuropathic osteoarthropathy. Furthermore, it will become even more important to identify the risk factors that are associated with the occurrence of this limb-threatening lower extremity complication.

Risk factors

Epidemiological studies are helpful with identifying the risk factors for Charcot neuroarthropathy. Potential risk factors associated with DNOAP in addition to neuropathy include age, sex, weight, duration with diabetes, and osteoporosis [12]. However, the ratio of men to women with Charcot arthropathy is approximately the same and no definite sex predilection has been recorded to date [17,28].

Age is an associated risk factor with neuropathic joint disease. When neuropathic osteoarthropathy is caused by a congenital indifference to pain or myelomeningocoele, the clinical presentation can occur in a child [12]. However, in patients with diabetes it typically presents during the fifth or sixth decade of life [29]. Other studies report the average age of diabetic neuropathic osteoarthropathy is approximately 57 years with most patients in their sixth and seventh decades [5,19].

Weight may be a considerable risk factor since the typical patient with diabetes-related Charcot arthropathy is overweight [30]. The mean body mass index (BMI) of Charcot patients according to Pakarinen and colleagues [24] was 32.9 kg/m^2 and 34.5 kg/m^2 in men and women, respectively.

Duration of diabetes may be an associated risk factor for the development of DNOAP. A review of 85 patients presenting with acute Charcot arthropathy revealed that there are type differences in the demographic features of patients with type 1 and type 2 diabetes developing acute Charcot [29]. Patients with type 1 had a longer duration of diabetes than that with type 2, but developed Charcot at an earlier age. Petrova and colleagues

[29] report that in patients with type 1 diabetes the most frequent decade of presentation is the fifth decade, while in type 2 it is in the sixth decade [29]. A long-standing history, at least a decade, with diabetes is common [5,17,31]. In type 1, the highest rate of presentation was among those with a 20- to 24-year duration of diabetes, while for type 2 the highest rate of presentation was with a 5- to 9-year duration. In another retrospective study of 36 patients with Charcot deformities, 41% of patients had type 1 diabetes and 59% had type 2 [24]. Eighty-eight percent of the patients required insulin for control of their diabetes and 12% were managed with diet or oral medication [24]. The average duration of type 1 was 28 years and type 2 was 14 years [24].

Peripheral neuropathy is associated with all disorders that produce neuro-arthropathy. Severe peripheral neuropathy typically creates a loss in protective sensation. Patients with diabetes frequently have a mixed neurological deficit with components of sensory, motor and/or autonomic neuropathy. A lack of sensory and proprioceptive awareness, sympathetic disinhibition from autonomic neuropathy, localized osteopenia, and continued weight bearing on unstable joints can lead to deterioration of the traumatic, arthritic, and/or avascular processes that occur with DNOAP [32]. In Fabrin and Holstein's study, 100% of patients had peripheral neuropathy as determined by clinical exam and biothesiometer [16]. The prevalence of peripheral polyneuropathy in the diabetic patient is estimated to be 9.00% to −32.00%, while that of Charcot neuroarthropathy in the overall diabetic population is estimated at 0.09% to 1.40% [24].

The relationship between bone mineral density (BMD) and Charcot arthropathy is unclear. It is unknown whether regional osteopenia is a risk factor for developing neuropathic joint disorders or is a result of the inflammatory process that accompanies the bone injury [33]. The osseous structures may be weakened as the result of hyperemic response, metabolic abnormalities, or periods of restricted weight bearing from other preexisting conditions. Nonetheless, osteopenia has been shown radiographically in severe neuropathy [34] and decreased bone mineral density with diabetic neuropathic osteoarthropathy [29,33,35,36]. Petrova and colleagues [36] measured the calcaneal bone density in type 1 and type 2 patients with unilateral Charcot deformities and those patients without the disorder. The calcaneal bone density in the Charcot foot was lower in both type 1 and type 2 diabetic patients [36]. It was also found that bone density was reduced in the non-Charcot foot in type 1 but not in type 2 patients [36].

Diabetic Charcot arthropathy of the foot and ankle also differs according to the pattern of initial destruction [33]. Herbst and colleagues [33] prospectively studied 55 patients with osteoarthropathy and used dual energy x-ray absorptiometry of the contralateral femoral neck or distal radius to evaluate peripheral bone density. Sixty-one Charcot feet or ankles were divided into three subtypes: fracture pattern, dislocation pattern, and combined fracture-dislocation pattern. The fracture pattern was associated with a peripheral deficiency of bone mineral density (BMD), while the dislocation pattern was associated with a normal BMD.

The common underlying factor in the development of Charcot arthropathy is a loss of protective sensation with continued weight bearing and repetitive stress applied to compromised joints in the foot and ankle [5,31]. The initial bone injury is usually subtle and unrecognized by the neuropathic patient. A history of an instigating event preceding the onset of a Charcot foot has been reported from 22% to 73% of the time [7,24,32]. For instance, Charcot arthropathy of the spine has occurred following traumatic paraplegia [37]. The literature also reports surgically induced Charcot arthropathy following podiatric, orthopedic, vascular, and transplantation surgery. Darst and colleagues [38] describe a case report of osteoarthropathy following a Keller arthroplasty for a recalcitrant hallux ulceration in diabetic patient with peripheral neuropathy. Zgonis and colleagues [39] report a case study of DNOAP following partial forefoot amputation. Last, Fishco [40] provides multiple case reports of Charcot joints developing in neuropathic feet following elective podiatric surgery.

An increased rate of DNOAP has been noted in simultaneous pancreas-kidney transplant patients. Flour reports 12% of 66 patients developed neuropathic jointspost-transplant; 4 of them presented within 1 year following transplantation [41]. Also in this study, four patients developed bilateral involvement at a mean of 1.4 ± 2.2 years. Interestingly, a mean pretransplant HbA1c was statistically greater in those patients who developed osteoarthropathy, and those with Charcot feet had an increased risk for rejection [41].

In summary, age, weight, duration of diabetes, peripheral neuropathy, decreased BMD, and a history of transplant surgery have been proposed as risk factors for developing DNOAP. Gender does not appear to be associated with the disorder. Table 3 presents characteristics of patients diagnosed with DNOAP from several selected studies.

Distribution of Charcot involvement

Neuropathic joint disease usually begins in a single joint and then progresses to involve other joints, depending on the underlying neurologic disorder and site of initial injury. Joint instability and subluxation occur as the disease progresses [12].

Although neuropathic osteoarthropathy most frequently affects the joints in the foot and ankle, there have been case reports of involvement in the shoulder [42,43], knee [44], and wrist [45]. In tabes dorsalis, knees, hips, and ankles are most commonly affected [12]. In syringomyelia, the glenohumeral joint, elbow, and wrist are commonly involved [12]. The most common presentation at this time is in patients with diabetes mellitus wherein the tarsometatarsal and tarsal joints are most commonly involved [12]. Less frequently, the ankle joint is affected, either alone or in concert with

Table 3
Patient characteristics with diabetic neuropathic osteoarthropathy

Reference	Average age (range)	Sex	Duration of diabetes
Sinha et al (1971)	2/3 in 50s to 60s (20–79)	58 M 43 F	66 patients > 15 y 35 patients 5–14 y
Cofield et al (1983)	56 (27–79)	N/A	81% > 10
Myerson et al (1994)	54 (25–73)	28 M 40 F	75% required insulin
Fabrin and Holstein (2000)	54 (27–80)	59 M 56 F	Type 1: 22 y (27–80) Type 2: 8 y (0–19) 82% of population IDDM
Pakarinen et al (2002)	51	22 M 10 F	IDDM: 28 y (8–58) 42% of population NIDDM: 14 y (1–28)
Herbst et al (2004)	Fracture pattern: 49.1 ± 15.6 y	15 M	Fracture pattern: 20 ± 12 y
	Dislocation pattern: 54.8 ± 9.1 y	31 F	Dislocation pattern: 21 ± 12 y
	Combined fracture-dislocations: 51.4 ± 10.9 y		Combined fracture-dislocation: 12 ± 8.5 y

Abbreviations: F, male; IDDM, insulin-dependent diabetes mellitus; M, male; N/A, not available; NIDDM, non–insulin-dependent diabetes mellitus.

other joints of the midfoot and rearfoot [46]. The typical patterns of involvement in the foot have been reported by several authors, with the most common being in the midfoot [5,33].

Sanders [5] and Frykberg provide a classification based on anatomic involvement in the foot and ankle. These patterns may occur individually or with multiple levels of involvement. Pattern one involves the forefoot and occurs in 15% of cases. Pattern two involves the tarsometatarsal joints and occurs in 40% in cases. Pattern three involves the midtarsal and naviculocuneiform joints and occurs in 30% of the cases. Pattern four involves the ankle and subtalar joints and occurs in 10% of reported cased. Last, Pattern five affects the calcaneus (calcaneal insufficiency avulsion fracture) in approximately 5% of cases [5].

The pattern of Charcot distribution in the Herbst [33] study included 19% ankles, 28% hindfeet, 50% midfeet, and 3% forefeet. In Pakarinen's study of 36 cases of diabetic Charcot arthropathy, the midfoot was involved in 86%, forefoot in 13.8%, ankle joint in 8.3%, and in the calcaneus in 2.7% of cases [24]. Schon's experience included 22.6% ankles, 10% hindfeet, 59.2% midfeet, and 8% forefeet (Table 4) [32].

The distribution of joint involvement depends on the underlying cause of the neurological deficit. While most frequently having a unilateral presentation, bilateral involvement has been reported to occur in 5.9% to 39.3% of cases [5,17]. Others have reported a much higher level of bilateral

Table 4
Distribution of involvement

Reference	Distribution
Sinha et al (1971)	12% ankle, 47% tarsal, 34% tarso-metatarsal, 34% metatarsophalangeal
Myerson et al (1994)	73% tarsometatarsal and naviculocuneiform, 27% talonavicular and calcanealcuboid
Schon et al (1998)	22.6% ankle, 10.0% hindfoot, 59.2% midfoot, 8.0% forefoot
Fabrin and Holstein (2000)	10/140 ankle, 26/140 forefoot,104/140 midfoot
Frykberg (2000)	10% ankle/subtalar, 5% calcaneus, 30% midtarsal, 40% tarsometatarsal, 15% forefoot
Pakarinen et al (2002)	8.3% ankle, 2.7% calcaneus, 86.0% midfoot, 13.8% forefoot
Herbst (2004)	19% ankle, 28% hindfoot, 50% midfoot, 3% forefoot
	23 with fracture pattern, 23 dislocation pattern and 9 patients with combination of fracture/dislocation

involvement, with radiographic changes noted in up to 75% of patients [47]. Young and colleagues [35] suggest that this is because of neurological deficits that are found symmetrically in diabetic patients Table 5.

Morbidity and mortality

Morbidity and mortality are related to the disease process and the cause of the disease and its related complications. Charcot neuroarthropathy has been recognized for over 130 years and yet it remains a major cause of morbidity for patients with diabetes mellitus. Two thirds of people with Charcot foot have type 2 diabetes [17,19,48]. Advances in medical treatment of diabetes have resulted in both an increased lifespan and improved quality of life for diabetic patients, but many have eventual problems with their feet [24]. The major morbidity of a Charcot joint is deformity from either an osseous prominence, "rocker bottom foot," or joint instability (especially noteworthy in the ankle) [9]. Deformity or instability can all to often lead to ulceration, infection, and ultimate amputation [46]. A recent benchmark analysis shows that diabetic patients with Charcot feet have especially high

Table 5
Percentage of bilateral involvement

Reference	Bilateral involvement, %
Sinha et al (1971)	23.7%
Myerson et al (1994)	31%
Fabrin and Holstein (2000)	17.9%
	1/140 simultaneous involvement
	24/140 nonsimultaneous involvement
Herbst (2004)	9.83%

morbidity, rates of hospitalization, and use of medical resources [31]. Further studies are needed assess the quality of life and working capacity of patients with DNOAP.

Globally, diabetes is the fifth leading cause of death [49]. Although increased morbidity is found in patients with Charcot deformity, an increased mortality rate in these patients has also been suggested. Gazi and colleagues [50] performed a comprehensive review of patients at the diabetic foot clinic at the City Hospital in Nottingham, UK. The survival and incidence of amputations in patients with diabetic neuropathic arthropathy was compared with those diabetic patients without Charcot involvement. According to this study, the mortality of diabetic patients with Charcot foot was just as high as those with neuropathic ulceration. In those patients with osteoarthropathy, 44.7% died after a mean of 3.7 years. Of particular note, 23.4% of patients with Charcot arthropathy required a major amputation, while only 10.6% of patients without this disorder succumbed to a major amputation [50].

Summary

According to the World Health Organization, the prevalence of diabetes worldwide is anticipated to increase from 171 million to 366 million by the year 2030 [51]. With this increase in diabetes, it is likely that foot and ankle specialists will encounter a greater number of Charcot foot presentations. Successful management of DNOAP is greatly facilitated when there is a heightened awareness of the pathogenesis, clinical presentation, natural history, predisposing risk factors, and common sites of involvement. Charcot ended his 1868 paper on tabetic arthropathies with the words "sera continue" ("to be continued") [11]. Early recognition and treatment are crucial in obtaining a satisfactory outcome. Perhaps further epidemiological studies will help clinicians identify populations at risk and individual risk factors, and develop evidence-based protocols to prevent or control the morbidity and mortality associated with DNOAP.

References

[1] Rockett I. Population and health: an introduction to epidemiology. Popul Bull 1999 cited 2007; Available at: http://findarticles com/p/articles/mi_qa3761/is_199912/ai_n8856519. Accessed July 7, 2007.

[2] Dirckx J. Stedman's concise medical dictionary for the health professions. In: Dirckx J, editor. Illustrated 4th edition. Baltimore: Lippincott Williams and Wilkins; 2001. p. 324.

[3] Rajbhandari SJ, Jenkins RC, Davies C, et al. Charcot neuroarthropathy in diabetes mellitus. Diabetologia 2002;45:1085–96.

[4] Frykberg RG, Mendeszoon E. Management of the diabetic Charcot foot. Diabetes Metab Res Rev 2000;16:S59–66.

[5] Sanders LF. Charcot neuroathropathy of the foot. In: Bowker J, Pfeifer M, editors. The diabetic foot. 6th edition. St. Louis: Mosby; 2001. p. 439–66.

[6] Sanders L, Frykberg R. Charcot neuroathropathy of the foot. In: Bowker J, Pfeifer M, editors. The Diabetic Foot. 6th edition. St. Louis: Mosby; 2001. p. 439–66.

[7] Cooper P. Application of external fixators for management of Charcot deformities of the foot and ankle. Foot Ankle Clin 2002;7:207–54.

[8] Chantelau E, Richter A, Ghassem-Zadeh N, et al. "Silent" bone stress injuries in the feet of diabetic patients with polyneuropathy: a report on 12 cases. Arch Orthop Trauma Surg 2007; 127(3):171–7.

[9] Armstrong D, Peters E. Charcot's arthropathy of the foot. International Diabetes Monitor 2001;13(5):1–5.

[10] Jeffcoate W, Lima J, Nobrega L. The Charcot foot. Diabet Med 1999;17:253–8.

[11] Sanders L. The Charcot foot: historical perspective 1827–2003. Diabetes Metab Res Rev 2004;20(1):S4–8.

[12] Gilliland B. Neuropathic joint disease in relapsing polychonditis and other arthritdes. 14th edition. Harrison's principles of internal medicine. In: Fauci A, Braunwald E, Isselbacher K, et al, editors. vol. 2. 1998, New York: McGraw-Hill; 1953.

[13] Mrugeshkumar S, Panis W. Neuropathic arthropathy (charcot joint). 2007. Available at: www.emedicine.com. Accessed July 7, 2007.

[14] Moonot PA, Ashwood N, Lockwood D. Orthopaedic complications of leprosy. J Bone Joint Surg [Br] 2005;87:1328–32.

[15] Cofield RH, Motrisin M, Beabout JW. Diabetic neuroarthropathy in the foot: patient characteristics and patterns of radiographic changes. Foot Ankle Int 1983;4:15–22.

[16] Fabrin J, Larsen K, Holstein P. Long-term follow-up in diabetic Charcot feet with spontaneous onset. Diabetes Care 2000;23:796–800.

[17] Hartemann-Heurtier A, Ha Van G, Grimaldi A. The Charcot foot. Lancet 2002;360:1776–9.

[18] Sella EJ, Barrette C. Staging of Charcot neuroarthropathy along the medial column of the foot in the diabetic patient. J Foot Ankle Surg 1999;38:34–40.

[19] Sinha S, Munichoodappa C, Kozak G. Neuro-arthropathy (Charcot joints) in diabetes mellitus. Medicine 1971;51:191–210.

[20] Foltz K, Fallat L, Schwartz S. Usefulness of a brief assessment battery for early dectection of Charcot foot deformity in patients with diabetes. J Foot Ankle Surg 2004;43(2):87–92.

[21] Marks R. Complications of foot and ankle surgery in patients with diabetes. Clin Orthop 2001;391:153–61.

[22] Myerson M, Henderson M, Saxby T, et al. Management of midfoot diabetic neuroarthropathy. Foot Ankle Int 1994;15(5):233–41.

[23] Chantelau E. The perils of procrastination: effects of early vs. delayed detection and treatment of incipient Charcot fracture. Diabet Med 2005;22(12):1707–12.

[24] Pakarinen T, Laine HJ, Honokonen SE, et al. Charcot arthropathy of the diabetic foot. Current concepts and review of 36 cases. Scand J Surg 2002;91(2):195–201.

[25] Gill G, Hayat H, Majid S. Diagnostic delays in diabetic Charcot arthropathy. Practical Diabetes International 2004;21(7):261–2.

[26] Lavery L, Armstrong D, Wunderlich R, et al. Diabetic foot syndome: evaluating the prevalence and incidence of foot pathology in Mexican Americans and non-Hispanic whites from a diabetes management cohort. Diabetes Care 2003;26:1435–8.

[27] McIntyre I, Boughen C, Trepman E, et al. Foot and ankle problems of aboriginal and non-aborginal diabetic patients with end-stage renal disease. Foot Ankle Int 2007;28(6):674–86.

[28] Mrugeshkumar S, Panis W. Neuropathic arthropathy (Charcot joint) 2007. Available at www.emedicine.com. Accessed July 7, 2007.

[29] Petrova N, Foster A, Edmunds M. Difference in presentation of Charcot osteoarthropathy in Type 1 compared with Type 2 Diabetes. Diabetes Care 2004;27(5):1235.

[30] Pinzur M. Benchmark analysis of diabetic patients with neuropathic (Charcot) foot deformity. Foot Ankle Int 1999;20(9):564–7.

[31] Lee L, Blume P, Sumpio B. Charcot joint disease in diabetes mellitus. Ann Vasc Surg 2003; 17:571–80.

[32] Schon L, Easley M, Weinfeld SB. Charcot neuorarthropathy of the foot and ankle. Clin Orthop 1998;349:116–31.
[33] Herbst S, Jones KB, Saltzman CL. Pattern of diabetic neuropathic arthropathy associated with the peripheral bone mineral density. J Bone Joint Surg [Br] 2004;86:378–83.
[34] Cundy T, Edmonds M, Watkins P. Osteopenia and metatarsal fractures in diabetic neuropathy. Diabet Med 1985;2:461–4.
[35] Young M, Marshall A, Adams J, et al. Osteopenia, neurological dysfunction, and the development of Charcot neuroarthropathy. Diabetes Care 1995;18(1):34–8.
[36] Petrova N, Foster AV, Edmunds ME. Calcaneal bone mineral density in patients with Charcot neuropathic osteoarthropathy: differences in Type 1 and Type 2 diabetes. Diabet Med 2005;22(6):756–61.
[37] Brown C, Jones B, Akmakijian J, et al. Neuropathic (Charcot) arthropathy of the spine after traumatic spinal paraplegia. Spine 1992;17(6):S103–8.
[38] Darst M, Weaver TD, Zangwill B. Charcot's joint following Keller arthroplasty. A case report. J Am Podiatr Med Assoc 1998;88(3):140–3.
[39] Zgonis T, Stapleton JJ, Shibuya N, et al. Surgically induced Charcot neuroarthropathy following partial forefoot amputation in diabetes. J Wound Care 2007;16(2):57–9.
[40] Fishco W. Surgically induced Charcot's foot. J Am Podiatr Med Assoc 2001;91(8):388–93.
[41] Flour M, Mathieu C. High rate of Charcot foot attacks early after simultaneous pancreas-kidney transplantation. Transplantation 2007;83(2):245–6.
[42] Edison J, Finger D. Neuropathic ostetoarthropathy of the shoulder. J Clin Rheumatol 2005;11(6):33–334.
[43] Jones J, Wolf S. Neuropathic shoulder arthropathy associated with syringomyelia. Neurology 1998;50(3):825–7.
[44] Lambert A, Close C. Charcot neuroarthropathy of the knee in Type 1 diabetes: treatment with total knee arthroplasty. Diabet Med 2002;19(4):338–41.
[45] Lambert A, Close C. Charcot neuroarthropathy of the wrist in type 1 diabetes. Diabetes Care 2005;28(4):984–5.
[46] Frykberg R, Zgonis T, Armstrong D, et al. Diabetic foot disorders. A clinical practice guideline (2006 revision). J Foot Ankle Surg 2006;45(5 Suppl):S1–66.
[47] Clohisy D, Thompson R. Fractures associated with neuropathic arthropathy in adults who have juvenile-onset diabetes. J Bone Joint Surg [Am] 1988;70:1192–6.
[48] Farber D, Juliano P, Cavanagh P, et al. Single stage correction with external fixation of the ulcerated foot in individuals with Charcot neuropathy. Foot Ankle Int 2002;23(2):130–4.
[49] Roglic G, Unwin N, Bennett P, et al. The burden of mortality attributable to diabetes: realistic estimates for the year 2000. Diabetes Care 2005;28:2130–5.
[50] Gazis A, Pound N, Macfarlane R, et al. Mortality in patients with diabetic neuropathy osteoarthropathy (Charcot foot). Diabet Med 2003;21:1243–6.
[51] WHO. Facts and figures on diabetes. World Health Oranization. 2007. Accessed July 7, 2007.

ELSEVIER
SAUNDERS

Clin Podiatr Med Surg
25 (2008) 29–42

CLINICS IN
PODIATRIC
MEDICINE AND
SURGERY

The Causes of the Charcot Syndrome

William Jeffcoate, MRCP

*Foot Ulcer Trials Unit, Department of Diabetes and Endocrinology Nottingham University
Hospitals Trust, City Hospital Campus, Nottingham, NG5 1PB, UK*

The hunt for the cause of what is often called "diabetic neuropathic osteoarthropathy" has been made difficult for several reasons. The first is that it is a condition without a definition. There are no specific pathologic markers of the disorder, and therefore no firm criteria on which the diagnosis may be based. This absence of a criterion standard means that the diagnosis rests essentially on pattern recognition, and pattern recognition itself is conditioned by the experience and beliefs of the clinician involved. Because the clinician relies on recognition of the association of nonspecific signs, the result is that some expert clinicians might make the diagnosis in instances when others might not, and this is especially true when the extent of damage is limited.

In addition, there is no experimental model available, and all theories concerning pathogenesis depend entirely on clinical observation of established cases. It can be difficult to determine which signs reflect an underlying predisposing cause and which are the consequence of the disease itself. This problem is compounded by the rarity of the disorder and the variation in clinical presentation. The third main reason is probably the most important, and this is the increasing realization that there is no single cause. Neuropathic osteoarthropathy occurs because of the varying and overlapping influences of factors that predispose to its development or make its occurrence unlikely. It is not a discrete disease in its own right but a process, a final common pathway.

That final common pathway does, however, have characteristic clinical features. In short, the acute syndrome is characterized by local inflammation that is associated with varying degrees of fracture and dislocation of bones and joints (in diabetes, this process is principally confined to the foot). The onset of the condition may be triggered by several different factors in an individual who is already at risk for one or more reasons, of which denervation is the most important. Finally, it is a disorder that is ultimately self-limiting,

E-mail address: wjeffcoate@futu.co.uk

0891-8422/08/$ - see front matter © 2008 Elsevier Inc. All rights reserved.
doi:10.1016/j.cpm.2007.10.003   *podiatric.theclinics.com*

reflecting the fact that it is essentially a functional abnormality that is caused by changes in the relative impact of different factors, even though these factors may themselves be irreversible. It is because this condition is not a discrete disease that the term *Charcot syndrome* is preferred.

Acute Charcot syndrome

Inflammation

The single most important clinical sign that underpins the diagnosis is the occurrence of local inflammation. If a foot is swollen but not warm, the diagnosis would not usually be considered. Indeed, inflammation may be the only sign if a case presents early, when plain radiographs may show no sign of skeletal damage. In such cases, it is necessary to establish that the inflammation is not confined to soft tissues (which may obviously result from unrelated disorders, such as infection or uncomplicated trauma), and this is best achieved by MRI or, with slightly less specificity, three-phase bone scan (see the article by Rogers and Bevilacqua elsewhere in this issue). It is the inflammation of bone that is associated with increasing bone lysis, which leads, in turn, to fracture and dislocation. As the disease settles, however, the signs of inflammation regress, and it is the absence of a temperature difference between the affected foot and the nonaffected foot that is the principal criterion used to allow the patient to start to resume weight bearing. It is only recently that it has been realized that the crucial part played by inflammation in clinical diagnosis and management simply reflects the important part played by inflammation in the evolution of the disease [1].

Role of proinflammatory cytokines

Experimental fracture in laboratory animals is associated with the acute-phase release of proinflammatory cytokines, including tumor necrosis factor-α (TNFα) and interleukin-1β (IL-1β) [2]. The expression of the proinflammatory cytokines, especially of TNFα, is closely associated with the increased expression of another cytokine system centered on the polypeptide, receptor activator of nuclear factor-κB (NF-κB) ligand (RANKL), which is a member of the TNF superfamily. RANKL is the ligand for the receptor activator of NF-κB (RANK) receptor, which, when activated, stimulates the formation of the nuclear transcription factor NF-κB. NF-κB has a variety of roles; however, when it is expressed in osteoclast precursor cells, it leads to their differentiation into mature osteoclasts, and hence to bone breakdown. Increased expression of the RANKL system has been shown to be associated in this way with the bone breakdown that occurs in many different circumstances, including osteoporosis (idiopathic, hypogonadal, or glucocorticoid induced), bone lysis caused by inflammation (rheumatoid arthritis, periodontitis, or prosthesis-related) or malignancy (especially myeloma), Paget's disease of bone, and other conditions [3–7].

Influence of reduced pain perception on the process of inflammation

It makes teleologic sense that fracture-induced inflammation leads to bone breakdown in this way, because one of the first stages of repair would involve the removal of bone fragments as a prelude to new bone formation [2,8–10]. After fracture, however, the process of inflammation is relatively short-lived and the increase in proinflammatory cytokines is greatest in the first 48 hours [2]. It is possible that this is because fracture is normally painful, and the pain leads to the broken bone being splinted. This, in turn, removes the stimulus to release of proinflammatory cytokines, and the process of inflammation is switched off [11]. When, however, a person has loss of pain perception as a result of nerve damage, the affected foot is not splinted in the same way; further trauma leads to further inflammation, and a vicious cycle is established. This leads to the progressive bone lysis that has been documented in Charcot syndrome [12–14], with increasing potential for fracture and dislocation while the condition remains active and untreated. The importance of splinting is reflected in the need for effective off-loading in management; off-loading serves not only to limit the forces applied to weakened bones but helps to abort the process of inflammation.

Predisposition

Denervation is currently thought to be an essential prerequisite for the development of the acute Charcot syndrome. The condition is rare, however, affecting perhaps only 1% of all people whose diabetes is complicated by neuropathy (see the article by Belczyk and Frykberg elsewhere in this issue). It follows that there must be factors other than neuropathy that put a person at risk.

Capacity to mount an inflammatory response

Absence of occlusive arterial disease

Because inflammation is central to the onset of the acute phase of the syndrome, it follows that one key permissive factor is the capacity to mount an inflammatory response.

It is probably for this reason that the acute Charcot syndrome is relatively uncommon in the elderly and in those with peripheral arterial disease: the mean age of presentation of 279 patients enrolled in a recent Internet-based survey was 57 years [15] and was 10 years younger than that in a unselected series of patients presenting with diabetic foot ulcers in the United Kingdom [16].

Retention of microvascular reactivity

Three groups have examined vascular reactivity in patients who had previously been diagnosed with Charcot syndrome and compared the findings with neuropathic controls [17–19]. All three groups reported that the skin of the foot of patients who had Charcot syndrome retained the capacity to vasodilate in response to warming, whereas that of neuropathic controls did not. This suggests that those who develop Charcot syndrome may have a specific, perhaps relatively limited, defect in neurovascular regulation and it is this that puts them at greater risk.

Premorbid hyperemia

One of the difficulties of having to base theories of cause on the clinical features at the time of presentation of the established syndrome is that it can be difficult to determine which features were present before the onset and might have played a causative role. Charcot himself noted the increase in blood flow at presentation and speculated that involvement of vasomotor nerves in the process of distal symmetric neuropathy might actually predispose to the onset of the syndrome by causing a defect of bone nutrition. Thus, he suggested that the hyperemia reflected an abnormality of bone blood flow that might cause bones to be "malnourished" in some way, and hence more liable to fracture (see panel) [20]:

> [Denervation] *devra se traduire encore par des troubles de la circulation ou de la nutrition, si elle affecte, en outre, des tubes appartenant au groupe des éléments nerveux vaso-moteurs ou trophiques* [denervation will also be expressed by changes in the circulation or nutrition if it involves, in addition, nerve fibers that are vasomotor or trophic].

Charcot was extraordinarily prescient in pinpointing the importance of abnormal vasomotor regulation but not, perhaps, completely correct in suggesting that this was linked to a preexisting weakness of bone. It is now known that distal symmetric neuropathy is indeed associated with increased flow of blood to the lower limb, and it results from decreased peripheral resistance and effective arteriovenous shunting, but the evidence that it is linked to reduced bone mineral density (BMD) is lacking. Moreover, hyperemia is a common feature of distal symmetric neuropathy (provided there is no associated occlusive arterial disease) [21], and this does not equate with the fact that the Charcot syndrome is so rare. Other observations also suggest that a neuropathy-related increase in premorbid blood flow is not a major causative factor. One is that the increased flow is symmetric, whereas the Charcot syndrome is usually asymmetric. Another is that the premorbid hyperemia is persistent, whereas the Charcot syndrome process eventually goes into remission. It is therefore likely that the hyperemia of underlying distal symmetric neuropathy may play a subtle part in the pathogenesis in some individuals but that in most cases, it is the further exaggeration of distal limb blood flow in the affected foot, which is triggered by an inflammatory stimulus, that is central to the progression of the disorder [1].

Premorbid osteopenia

There have been several studies of BMD in diabetes, and the general conclusion is that there may be a tendency to osteopenia of the axial and distal skeleton in diabetes but that it is not marked and is, moreover, much more apparent in type 1 disease. Having said that, there is rather stronger evidence that osteopenia does occur when diabetes is complicated by neuropathy [22–25], and this seems to be equally prevalent in type 1 and type 2 disease [26]. It is therefore possible (although it is not clearly established) that although premorbid osteopenia is not a major causative factor, it might still be important in certain patient groups. Such groups might include that in which acute Charcot syndrome seems to be rather more common: those patients who have had a renal transplant. The preceding renal failure would have been associated with bone loss from vitamin D deficiency and hyperparathyroidism, and it may have been worsened after immunosuppression with glucocorticoids.

Another rare group in which premorbid osteopenia is especially likely to play a part is in the occasional patient (usually female) who presents with acute Charcot syndrome in the late teens or early twenties. This presentation typically follows the association of poor glycemic control with an eating disorder, and it is presumed that the typical reduction in BMD observed in teenagers (especially girls) with type 1 diabetes [27] is made worse by malnutrition.

Premorbid osteopenia may be important in those with vitamin D deficiency but without renal failure. Jirkovska and colleagues [28] have drawn attention to the possibility that vitamin D concentration may tend to be lower on average (and parathyroid hormone [PTH] higher on average) in those with Charcot syndrome. Such an effect may also underlie the known association between Charcot syndrome and nephropathy and may also be one factor that may underlie the suggestion that the prevalence of the disorder varies from country to country, with an unconfirmed suggestion that it is more common in colder climates. Whatever the significance of premorbid osteopenia, there is no doubt that once the disease is established, bone density decreases rapidly in the affected foot and, to a lesser extent, in the contralateral limb [13,14]. It is not known whether this contralateral osteopenia may be a causative factor in the 20% of patients who go on to get acute Charcot syndrome in the other foot.

Arterial calcification

The term *arterial calcification* is a misnomer because the process is actually one of ossification, but it is used here because it is conventional.

Such calcification of the arterial cell wall in diabetes usually takes the form of classic "pipe-stem" or Mönckeberg's sclerosis, which is visible on radiographs as parallel lines in arteries in profile or as rings in those that are end-on. The prevalence of such calcification has been reported to be of the order of 20% in diabetes without neuropathy [29] but rather higher in neuropathy [29–33]. Calcification also occurs in those with neuropathy complicating other diseases, but the prevalence is rather lower than in those with diabetes and neuropathy [32]. In Charcot syndrome, however, the reported prevalence is high, being of the order of 78% to 90% [34,35]. In some respects, this echoes the situation described previously with relevance to hyperemia; it is increased in those who may be predisposed to acute Charcot syndrome but worsens once the disease process is triggered. It is, however, not immediately clear whether calcification of the arterial wall actually causes or promotes the development of acute Charcot syndrome disease, even though the associated loss of compliance of the arterial wall results in an increase in arterial pulse pressure—a pulse pressure that is already widened as a result of decreased peripheral arterial resistance. This may lead to reduction of bone strength as a result of widened Haversian canals, as described many years ago in Charcot syndrome complicating syphilis [36]. Although this change in hemodynamics may play a part, it is perhaps more likely that the increasing prevalence of calcification is an epiphenomenon—a consequence of the change inherent in the development of the foot affected by Charcot syndrome and not a direct cause.

Even if increased calcification of the arterial wall is merely an epiphenomenon, it might offer a clue to the processes involved in the predisposition to, and progression of the disorder. It is relevant that the significance of calcification, osteopenia, and blood flow is similar in that they are all features of neuropathy in diabetes and all of them become exaggerated once the Charcot syndrome process becomes established. They are also linked by their dependence on the RANKL/osteoprotegerin (OPG) cytokine system.

Receptor activator of nuclear factor-κB ligand/osteoprotegerin cytokine system

The key part played by the RANKL/OPG cytokine system is the subject of the unifying hypothesis that has been proposed for the evolution of Charcot syndrome [1]. There is no direct evidence of its involvement, but the circumstantial evidence is strong.

Receptor activator of nuclear factor-κB ligand/osteoprotegerin system

RANKL may be expressed by a variety of cells, including macrophages and osteoclast precursors. It is the ligand for the RANK receptor, which, when activated, leads to expression of the nuclear transcription factor NF-κB [3–7]. One of the actions of NF-κB is to increase the expression of the glycoprotein OPG, which is structurally similar to the RANK receptor and serves as a decoy receptor for RANKL. Any increase in the expression of RANKL is therefore linked to an increase in OPG, and OPG effectively antagonizes or neutralizes its effects. It follows that the two cytokines are elevated in the same clinical circumstances, even though their effects are opposite. This means that it can be difficult to assess causative relations when increased expression of either is demonstrated in different clinical circumstances. Nevertheless, it is becoming increasingly apparent that the

RANKL/OPG system is central to many pathophysiologic processes of arteries and bone. Needless to say, such a basic mechanism is necessarily subject to a variety of regulatory mechanisms, including those that enhance the expression of RANKL (eg, PTH, glucocorticoids, TNFα) and those that inhibit it (including sex steroids, calcitonin, and calcitonin gene-related peptide [CGRP]). It may also be modulated by leptin and by islet amyloid polypeptide (IAPP) (Fig. 1) [1]. The expression of RANKL may also be increased by ambient glucose, hyperlipidemia, and advanced glycation end products (AGEs).

Receptor activator of nuclear factor-κB ligand and osteoprotegerin in mediating inflammation

The acute Charcot syndrome is essentially an inflammatory arthropathy, and, as described previously, any acute inflammation is mediated by the release of proinflammatory cytokines, including TNFα. The functional relation between TNFα and RANKL is close and complex, but RANKL expression increases at the onset of inflammation.

Receptor activator of nuclear factor-κB ligand and osteoprotegerin involvement in osteolysis

The involvement of this cytokine system in bone breakdown has been outlined previously in this article. Whatever the significance of premorbid osteopenia, bone breakdown is accelerated once the Charcot syndrome process is initiated and a reinforcing cycle of inflammation is established. The inflammation is associated with increased expression of RANKL, and RANKL stimulates maturation of osteoclasts, leading to osteolysis and fracture.

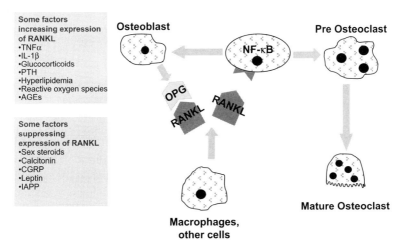

Fig. 1. Schematic representation of the RANKL/OPG cytokine system and some factors that modulate its expression. AGEs, advanced glycation end products.

Receptor activator of nuclear factor-κB ligand and osteoprotegerin in vascular calcification

There is increasing evidence that increased expression of RANKL (with or without TNFα) stimulates arterial calcification by inducing the apoptosis of vascular smooth muscle cells and by causing the differentiation of precursor cells (pericytes, vascular smooth muscle cells, and adventitial cells) into cells with osteogenic potential [36–41]. Once they develop into bone-forming cells, they acquire the capacity to express OPG, which serves, presumably, to dampen the process.

Receptor activator of nuclear factor-κB ligand and osteoprotegerin in diabetes

Serum concentrations of OPG (and hence, presumably, of RANKL, which is less commonly studied because it is less easy to measure) are elevated in diabetes, unrelated to the Charcot syndrome. In children with diabetes and in adults with newly diagnosed type 1 diabetes, the increase in OPG correlates directly with the quality of blood glucose control [42,43]. In those with more established disease, the elevation in OPG seems to correlate more closely with disease duration [44,45]. It is also known that RANKL expression is increased by free radicals [46], hyperlipidemia [47], mean glucose concentration [48], and AGEs [49].

Receptor activator of nuclear factor-κB ligand and osteoprotegerin in neuropathy in diabetes

An association has also been demonstrated between circulating concentrations of OPG and the presence of nephropathy and retinopathy in diabetes [45], even though none has so far been sought with neuropathy, with which nephropathy and retinopathy are commonly associated. If an association between neuropathy and increased expression of RANKL is confirmed, it is possible that it is mediated by means of the loss of neuropeptides normally elaborated in nerve terminals, such as CGRP and substance P (see Fig. 1) [50,51]. It has been argued that activation of the RANKL/OPG system could therefore be the key to the association between neuropathy and arterial calcification [52].

Receptor activator of nuclear factor-κB ligand and osteoprotegerin and changes in bone density in diabetes

One study has reported an association between OPG and BMD in children with type 1 diabetes [42], and another has reported as association with circulating concentrations of bone turnover markers in men with type 2 disease [53]. No correlation between OPG and BMD was, however, found in a large cohort of adult women with and without type 2 disease [54]. It should be noted, however, that type 2 diabetes, which is not complicated by neuropathy, is not generally thought to be associated with osteopenia; thus, the lack of any strong association with circulating OPG in this study is not altogether surprising. It is not known whether this is associated with increased expression of the RANKL/OPG system.

Receptor activator of nuclear factor-κB ligand and osteoprotegerin and vascular calcification in diabetes

Several groups have shown that increased calcification of the coronary arteries is independently associated with increased circulating concentrations of OPG in diabetes [55–57], and concentrations of OPG are also known to be independently associated with prior [58] and future [54,57] cardiovascular disease.

Unifying hypothesis concerning the role of the receptor activator of nuclear factor-κB ligand/osteoprotegerin in the pathogenesis of the acute Charcot syndrome in diabetes

Receptor activator of nuclear factor-κB ligand and osteoprotegerin in the person at risk for Charcot syndrome

It is thought that a person is predisposed to the development of Charcot syndrome by having diabetes, neuropathy, and the capacity to mount an inflammatory reaction in the foot. Although much of the available evidence is circumstantial, it strongly suggests that such an at-risk group may also be characterized by increased expression of RANKL. Increased expression of RANKL or OPG is observed in diabetes and especially in diabetes complicated by other microvascular complications. Although there are no data to prove a link with distal symmetric neuropathy, there is evidence of associations between RANKL/OPG activation and osteopenia and vascular calcification, each of which is closely associated with neuropathy.

Receptor activator of nuclear factor-κB ligand and osteoprotegerin in the active phase of acute Charcot syndrome

The factor that probably initiates most cases of acute Charcot syndrome is an external stimulus that causes localized inflammation, as described previously, and the process enters a vicious cycle of augmentation because loss of protective sensation inhibits effective immobilization. It is known that the process of acute inflammation is associated with increased expression of RANKL, and it is therefore probable that the syndrome occurs in this at-risk group because the resultant effect on bone breakdown (leading to fracture and dislocation) is greatest in those in whom RANKL expression may already be rather high.

Genetic predisposition

It is possible that some people have a genetic predisposition to develop acute Charcot syndrome. In this respect, the Charcot syndrome might resemble Paget's disease of bone, in which a variety of polymorphisms have been identified, including those that have an impact on the RANKL/OPG system [59]. To date, however, this possibility has not been investigated.

Spectrum of Charcot syndrome in diabetes

The number of factors that may be involved in determining the extent and duration of increased expression of RANKL-induced osteolysis goes some way toward explaining the variation observed in the presentation of the acute foot affected by Charcot syndrome in diabetes. It is possible that the degree of sensory loss is important, and Kimmerle and Chantelau [60] have recently reported that those who have continued to take weight on the affected foot (and are thus likely to be those who feel less pain) have more extensive deformity. Herbst and colleagues [61] have suggested that the extent of osteopenia at the time of presentation is also reflected in the relative prevalence of fracture and dislocation, with fracture being more common in those with reduced bone density. Individual factors also provide some explanation for the increased incidence in certain particularly vulnerable groups, such as those with vitamin D deficiency, those who have had a renal transplant, or young women with a history of an eating disorder.

Differences between Charcot syndrome in diabetes and other disease

Consideration of the spectrum of factors that might predispose to the development of the syndrome invites novel speculation on factors that determine the presentation of Charcot syndrome in disease other than diabetes. The other condition in which it is most often observed in Western countries is neuropathy associated with alcohol abuse, in which the presentation is similar to that observed in diabetes. Although alcohol abuse is more closely associated with osteopenia than is diabetes, the presentation is otherwise similar and the pathogenesis is likely to be related simply to the distal symmetric neuropathy. Because neuropathy is worst in the extremities, it explains why foot involvement is more common in these disorders. The neuropathy associated with leprosy is, however, infective rather than toxic; hence, joint involvement is not necessarily so peripheral. In tabes dorsalis, however, Charcot syndrome most typically affects the large joints, and it is possible that this is because loss of deep pain sensation is much more profound in this condition. It is also possible that the associated loss of proprioception in tabes dorsalis predisposes to damage to the larger joints through abnormalities of gait. Finally, traumatic denervation is also associated with loss of sensation, which is likely to be near total, and with motor neuropathy and hypotonia, which increase the risk for dislocation.

Summary

The term *Charcot syndrome* is suggested because the disorder is not a single disorder but a complex of changes occurring in individuals who are predisposed to its development by several different overlapping factors occurring in several different diseases. In the case of the diabetic foot, the main predisposing factors are the presence of diabetes itself, combined with neuropathy and with preservation of the peripheral circulation. The condition only occurs when an unrelated event triggers the onset of inflammation in the affected foot, however. Instead of being short-lived, this inflammation becomes protracted as a direct result of lost protective sensation and failure to immobilize the limb. As the inflammatory phase persists, there is progressive osteolysis and damage to the bones and joints. It is further suggested that the person with diabetes and neuropathy is predisposed by increased expression of RANKL and that this expression is increased further by the advent of inflammation. The increased expression of RANKL explains the worsening osteopenia that is observed as the disease progresses and the high prevalence of vascular calcification observed in those who have had it.

References

[1] Jeffcoate WJ, Game FL, Cavanagh PR. The role of proinflammatory cytokines in the cause of neuropathic osteoarthropathy (acute Charcot foot) in diabetes. Lancet 2005;366:2058–61.

[2] Kon T, Cho TJ, Aizawa T, et al. Expression of osteoprotegerin, receptor activator of NF-kappaB ligand (osteoprotegerin ligand) and related proinflammatory cytokines during fracture healing. J Bone Miner Res 2001;16:1004–14.

[3] Khosla S. Minireview: the OPG/RANK system. Endocrinology 2001;142:5050–5.

[4] Hofbauer LC, Schoppet M. Osteoprotegerin: a link between osteoporosis and arterial calcification? Lancet 2001;358:257–9.

[5] Boyle WJ, Simonet WS, Lacey DL. Osteoclast differentiation and activation. Nature 2003; 423:337–42.

[6] Hofbauer LC, Schoppet M. Clinical implications of the osteoprotegerin/RANKL/RANK system for bone and vascular diseases. J Am Med Assoc 2004;292:490–5.

[7] Rogers A, Eastell R. Circulating osteoprotegerin and receptor activator for nuclear factor-kappaB ligand: clinical utility in metabolic bone disease assessment. J Clin Endocrinol Metab 2005;90:6323–31.

[8] Gerstenfeld LC, Cho TJ, Kon T, et al. Impaired intramembranous bone formation during bone repair in the absence of tumor necrosis factor-alpha signalling. Cells Tissues Organs 2001;169:285–94.

[9] Saidenberg-Kermanac'h N, Bessis N, Cohen-Salal M, et al. Osteoprotegerin and inflammation. Eur Cytokine Netw 2002;13:144–53.

[10] Lam J, Abu-Amer Y, Nelson CA, et al. Tumour necrosis factor superfamily cytokines and the pathogenesis of inflammatory osteolysis. Ann Rheum Dis 2002;61:82–3.

[11] Sugawara J, Hayashi K, Kaneko F, et al. Reductions in basal limb blood flow and lumen diameter after short-term leg casting. Med Sci Sports Exerc 2004;36:1689–94.

[12] Petrova NL, Foster AV, Edmonds ME. Calcaneal bone mineral density in patients with Charcot neuropathic osteoarthropathy: differences between Type 1 and Type 2 diabetes. Diabet Med 2005;22(6):756–61.

[13] Jirkowská A, Kasalický P, Boucek P, et al. Calcaneal ultrasonometry in patients with Charcot osteoarthropathy and its relationship with densitometry in the lumbar spine and femoral neck and with markers of bone turnover. Diabet Med 2001;18(6):495–500.

[14] Hastings MK, Sinacore DR, Fielder FA, et al. Bone mineral density during total contact cast immobilization for a patient with neuropathic (Charcot) arthropathy. Phys Ther 2005;85(3): 249–56.

[15] Game F, Catlow R, Jeffcoate W, et al. CDUK: a UK-wide, web-based survey of the management of the acute Charcot foot of diabetes. Diabetologia 2007;50(Suppl 1):P1116.

[16] Jeffcoate WJ, Chipchase SY, Ince P, et al. Assessing the outcome of the management of diabetic foot ulcers using ulcer-related and person-related measures. Diabetes Care 2006; 29(8):1784–7.

[17] Shapiro SA, Stansberry KB, Hill MA, et al. Normal blood flow response and vasomotion in the diabetic Charcot foot. J Diabetes Complications 1998;12:147–53.

[18] Veves A, Akbari CM, Primavera J, et al. Endothelial dysfunction and the expression of endothelial nitric oxide synthetase in diabetic neuropathy, vascular disease, and foot ulceration. Diabetes 1998;47:457–63.

[19] Baker N, Green A, Krishnan S, et al. Microvascular and C-fiber function in diabetic Charcot neuro-arthropathy and diabetic peripheral neuropathy. Diabetes Care 2007;30(12): 3077–9.

[20] Charcot JM. Sur quelques arthropathies qui paraiise dépendre d'une lésion du cerveau ou de la mouelle épinière. Arch Physiol Norm Pathlo 1868;1:161–78.

[21] Edmonds ME, Roberts VC, Watkins PJ. Blood flow in the diabetic neuropathic foot. Diabetologia 1982;22(1):9–15.

[22] Cundy T, Edmonds ME, Watkins PJ. Osteopenia and metatarsal fractures in diabetic neuropathy. Diabet Med 1985;2:461–4.

[23] Kayath MJ, Dib SA, Viela JG. Prevalence and magnitude of osteopenia associated with insulin-dependent diabetes mellitus. J Diabetes Complications 1994;8:97–104.

[24] Forst T, Pfutzner A, Kann P, et al. Peripheral osteopenia in adult patients with insulin-dependent diabetes mellitus. Diabet Med 1995;12:874–9.

[25] Rix M, Andreasson H, Eskilden P. Impact of peripheral neuropathy on bone density in patients with type 1 diabetes. Diabetes Care 1999;22:827–31.

[26] Ziegler R. Diabetes mellitus and bone metabolism. Horm Metab Res Suppl 1992;26:90–4.

[27] Léger J, Marinovic D, Alberti C, et al. Lower bone mineral content in children with type 1 diabetes mellitus is linked to female sex, low insulin-like growth factor type I levels, and high insulin requirement. J Clin Endocrinol Metab 2006;91(10):3947–53.

[28] Jirkovska A, Bém R, Fejfarová V, et al. Longitudinal study of vitamin D insufficiency and its association with osteoclastic activity in patients with Charcot osteoarthropathy. Diabetes 2007;55(Suppl 1):260, 0R.

[29] Psyrogiannis A, Kyriazooulou V, Vagenakis AG. Medial arterial calcification is frequently found in patients with microalbuminuria. Angiology 1999;50:971–5.

[30] Whitehouse FW, Weckstein M. On diabetic osteopathy: a radiographic study of 21 patients. Diabetes Care 1978;1:303–4.

[31] Edmonds ME, Morrison N, Laws JW, et al. Medial arterial calcification and diabetic neuropathy. Br Med J 1982;284:928–30.

[32] Lithner F, Hietala SO, Steen L. Skeletal lesions and arterial calcifications of the feet in diabetics. Acta Med Scand Suppl 1984;687:47–54.

[33] Gentile S, Bizarro A, Marmo R, et al. Medial arterial calcification and diabetic neuropathy. Acta Diabetol Lat 1990;27:243–53.

[34] Sinha S, Munichoodappa C, Kozak GP. Neuro-arthropathy (Charcot joints) in diabetes mellitus: a clinical study of 101 cases. Medicine (Baltimore) 1972;51:191–210.

[35] Clouse ME, Gramm HF, Legg M, et al. Diabetic osteoarthropathy: clinical and roentgenographic observations in 90 cases. Am J Roentgenol Radium Ther Nucl Med 1974;121:22–33.

[36] Knaggs RI. Charcot joints. In: Knaggs RI, editor. Inflammatory and toxic disorders of bone. Bristol (RI): John Wright & Sons; 1926. p. 105–19.

[37] Schoppet M, Al-Fakhri N, Franke FE, et al. Localization of osteoprotegerin, tumor necrosis factor-related apoptosis-inducing ligand, and receptor activator of nuclear factor-κB ligand in Mönckeberg's sclerosis and atherosclerosis. J Clin Endocrinol Metab 2004;89: 4104–12.

[38] Abedin M, Tintut Y, Demer LL. Vascular calcification. Arterioscler Thromb Vasc Biol 2004; 24:1161–70.

[39] Collin-Osdoby P. Regulation of vascular calcification by osteoclast regulatory factors RANKL and osteoprotegerin. Circ Res 2004;95:1046–57.

[40] Hruska KA, Mathew S, Saab G. Bone morphogenetic proteins in vascular calcification. Circ Res 2005;97(2):105–14.

[41] Hayden MR, Tyagi SC, Kolb L, et al. Vascular ossification-calcification in metabolic syndrome, type 2 diabetes mellitus, chronic kidney disease, and calciphylaxis-calcific ure-mic arteriolopathy: the emerging role of sodium thiosulfate. Cardiovasc Diabetol 2005; 4(1):4.

[42] Galluzzi F, Stagi S, Salti R. Osteoprotegerin serum levels in children with type 1 diabetes: a potential modulating role in bone status. Eur J Endocrinol 2005;153(6):879–85.

[43] Xiang GD, Sun HL, Zhao LS. Changes of osteoprotegerin before and after insulin therapy in type 1 diabetic patients. Diabetes Res Clin Pract 2007;76(2):199–206.

[44] Secchiero P, Corallini F, Pandolfi A, et al. An increased osteoprotegerin serum release char-acterizes the early onset of diabetes mellitus and may contribute to endothelial cell dysfunc-tion. Am J Pathol 2006;169(6):2236–44.

[45] Knudsen ST, Foss CH, Poulsen PL, et al. Increased plasma concentrations of osteoprote-gerin in type 2 diabetic patients with microvascular complications. Eur J Endocrinol 2003; 49(1):39–42.

[46] Jiang MZ, Tsukara H, Ohshima Y, et al. Effects of antioxidants and nitric oxide on TNF-alpha-induced adhesion molecule expression and NK-kappaB activation in human dermal microvascular endothelial cells. Life Sci 2004;75:1159–70.

[47] Tintut Y, Morony S, Demer LL. Hyperlipidemia promotes osteoclastic potential of bone marrow cells ex vivo. Arterioscler Thromb Vasc Biol 2004;e6–10.

[48] Yerneni KK, Rai W, Khan BV, et al. Hyperglycemia-induced activation of the transcription nuclear factor-kappaB in vascular smooth muscle cells. Diabetes 1999;48:855–64.

[49] Bierhaus A, Schiekofer S, Schwaninger M, et al. Diabetes-associated sustained activation of the transcription nuclear factor-kappaB. Diabetes 2001;50:2792–808.

[50] Imai S, Matsue Y. Neuronal regulation of bone metabolism and anabolism: calcitonin gene-related peptide-, substance P-, and tyrosine hydroxylase-containing nerves and the bone. Microsc Res Tech 2002;58:61–9.

[51] Ishizuka K, Hirukawa K, Nakamura H, et al. Inhibitory effect of CGRP on osteoclast formation by mouse bone marrow cells treated with isoproterenol. Neurosci Lett 2005; 379(1):47–51.

[52] Jeffcoate W. Vascular calcification and osteolysis in diabetic neuropathy—is RANK-L the missing link? Diabetologia 2004;47(9):1488–92.

[53] Suzuki K, Kurose T, Takizawa M, et al. Osteoclastic function is accelerated in male patients with type 2 diabetes mellitus: the preventive role of osteoclastogenesis inhibitory factor/osteoprotegerin (OCIF/OPG) on the decrease of bone mineral density. Diabetes Res Clin Pract 2005;68(2):117–25.

[54] Browner WS, Lui LY, Cummings SR. Associations of serum osteoprotegerin levels with diabetes, stroke, bone density, fractures, and mortality in elderly women. J Clin Endocrinol Metab 2001;86(2):631–7.

[55] Schoppet M, Sattler AM, Schaefer JR, et al. Increased osteoprotegerin serum levels in men with coronary artery disease. J Clin Endocrinol Metab 2003;88(3):1024–8.

[56] Avignon A, Sultan A, Piot C, et al. Osteoprotegerin is associated with silent coronary artery disease in high-risk but asymptomatic type 2 diabetic patients. Diabetes Care 2005;28(9): 2176–80.

[57] Anand DV, Lahiri A, Lim E, et al. The relationship between plasma osteoprotegerin levels and coronary artery calcification in uncomplicated type 2 diabetic subjects. J Am Coll Cardiol 2006;47(9):1850–7.

[58] Rasmussen LM, Tarnow L, Hansen TK, et al. Plasma osteoprotegerin levels are associated with glycaemic status, systolic blood pressure, kidney function and cardiovascular morbidity in type 1 diabetic patients. Eur J Endocrinol 2006;154(1):75–81.

[59] Daroszewska A, Ralston SH. Genetics of Paget's disease of bone. Clin Sci 2005;109(3): 257–63.

[60] Kimmerle R, Chantelau E. Weight-bearing intensity produces Charcot deformity in injured neuropathic feet in diabetes. Exp Clin Endocrinol Diabetes 2007;115(6):360–4.

[61] Herbst SA, Jones JB, Saltzman CL. Pattern of diabetic neuropathic arthropathy associated with the peripheral bone mineral density. J Bone Joint Surg 2004;86(3):378–83.

ELSEVIER
SAUNDERS

Clin Podiatr Med Surg
25 (2008) 43–51

CLINICS IN
PODIATRIC
MEDICINE AND
SURGERY

The Diagnosis of Charcot Foot

Lee C. Rogers, DPM*, Nicholas J. Bevilacqua, DPM

*Foot and Ankle Surgery, Amputation Prevention Center, Broadlawns Medical Center,
1801 Hickman Road, Des Moines, IA 50314 USA*

The diagnosis of Charcot foot is challenging, especially in its earliest stages. It is frequently misdiagnosed as cellulitis, deep venous thrombosis, or acute gout. In the later stages, when bone destruction is visible by radiography, it is commonly misdiagnosed as osteomyelitis. This can be particularly troublesome as it may lead some physicians to place patients on long-term antibiotics unnecessarily or recommend amputation as a treatment. The diagnostic delay averages 29 weeks [1], allowing insensate patients to cause continued trauma to the foot, worsening the deformity. Early detection and treatment can minimize fractures and incapacitating deformities [2]. Tan and colleagues [3] proposed that acute Charcot joint disease is a "medical emergency," as there are therapies available that can alter its natural history. The diagnosis of Charcot foot is made on clinical examination and imaging. Each is discussed below.

Clinical presentation

It has often been said that one must have a "high index of suspicion" for Charcot foot in those with diabetes, neuropathy, and a warm, swollen foot. The foot may appear to be edematous, erythematous, and can be palpably warmer than the contralateral side (Fig. 1). More advanced presentations of the disease may have obvious deformity, including the "rocker-bottom" deformity that is a hallmark of Charcot foot (Fig. 2A). Those with rocker-bottom deformities may have a plantar ulcer or a pre-ulcer under the focal point of plantar pressure (Fig. 2B). More than half of patients suffering from Charcot foot remember some incipient trauma, which to the patient could be trivial [4]. Some patients will report pain, even though peripheral neuropathy is evident on examination.

* Corresponding author.
E-mail address: lee.c.rogers@gmail.com (L.C. Rogers).

0891-8422/08/$ - see front matter © 2008 Elsevier Inc. All rights reserved.
doi:10.1016/j.cpm.2007.10.006
podiatric.theclinics.com

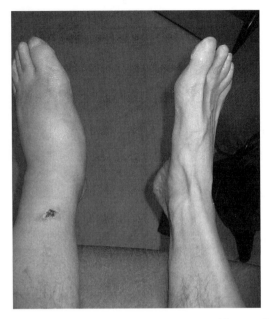

Fig. 1. A dorsal comparison view of the feet in a patient with acute Charcot foot.

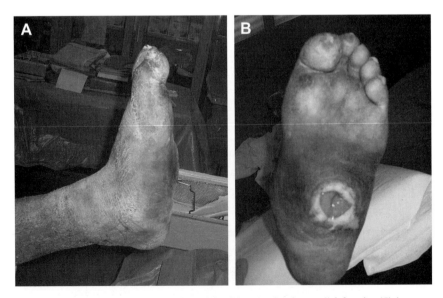

Fig. 2. (*A*) A medial view of a Charcot foot with evident "rocker-bottom" deformity. (*B*) A neuro-pathic ulcer on the plantar midfoot, typical of a rocker-bottom deformity.

Neuropathy is necessary for the onset of Charcot foot and can be confirmed by Semmes-Weinstein monofilament [4] or vibratory perception threshold [5]. Autonomic neuropathy is thought play a central role in the pathophysiology of Charcot foot and can be investigated clinically measuring heart rate variability (HRV) with deep breathing or orthostatic blood pressure. Stevens and colleagues [5] found a decrease in HRV and a postural fall in blood pressure in patients with Charcot foot and in diabetic individuals with ulcerated feet when compared with diabetic controls. HRV can be discovered by palpating the radial pulse while the patient inspires deeply and expires slowly. With an intact vagal response, the pulse will increase with inspiration and decrease with expiration, also termed physiologic arrhythmia. In those with cardiac autonomic neuropathy, the pulse rate will vary little or remain constant throughout the respiratory cycle.

Generally, the acute Charcot foot has no impairment of circulation, unlike other diabetic foot syndromes. Pedal pulses may be bounding in acute Charcot foot. Skin temperature difference between feet, as measured with a contact [6] or noncontact [7] thermometer, may be significant (Fig. 3). The average difference between the acute Charcot foot and the unaffected side is as much as 9°F. A difference of 4°F is considered significant [8].

Equinus contributes to the pathogenesis of Charcot arthropathy of the midfoot and is almost uniformly present in these cases. Many times, the equinus contracture is so advanced that the calcaneal inclination angle is a negative value on a weight-bearing lateral foot radiograph (Fig. 4).

Imaging of Charcot foot

Once the clinical exam causes one to suspect Charcot foot, the diagnosis will need to be confirmed with imaging. Plain radiographs are valuable in the diagnosis of Charcot foot, but even more so for the monitoring of the disease process. Eichenholtz [9] originally classified Charcot foot

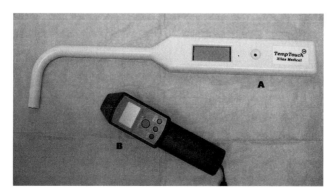

Fig. 3. Contact (A) and noncontact (B) thermometers.

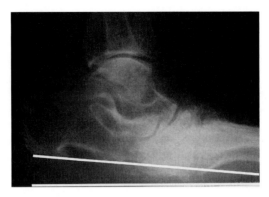

Fig. 4. A lateral radiograph of a foot with Charcot foot and severe equinus deformity. Note the negative calcaneal inclination angle.

radiographically with three stages. He describes Stage I (Stage of Development) as subchondral fragmentation and debris formation on radiograph. Stage II (Stage of Coalescense) is characterized by absorption of the fine debris, fusing of the larger fragments, and sclerosis of the bone ends. Stage III (Stage of Reconstruction) is marked by the bone ends and major fragments becoming "rounded" and some restoration of joint architecture may be seen.

Fig. 5 illustrates an algorithm for the use of imaging to diagnose Charcot foot. It is important to note that clinical correlation is implied in this algorithm by including "clinical suspicion" and the presence of an "open wound." If bone destruction is evident on radiograph, there is no need to perform a three-phase [99]Technetium (^{99}Tc) bone scan, as this is a nonspecific test and will be positive with any number of bone diseases. In the case where bone destruction is evident and there is no history of an open wound, one can be fairly confident that osteomyelitis is not present, as this would be very rare in cases with no portal of infection. These cases will most commonly be Charcot foot. If there is bone destruction *and* an open wound, osteomyelitis will have to be ruled out. Using a leukocyte-labeled bone scan ([111]Indium or [99m]Technetium hexamethylpropyleneamine oxime, HMPAO), one can exclude osteomyelitis (Fig. 6A, B) [10,11]. While some authors tout the ability of MRI to differentiate between Charcot foot and osteomyelitis [12], others cite that there is little difference [13]. If MRI is to be used, a few caveats should be remembered that can improve your sensitivity. Charcot foot is most common at the midfoot and commonly causes joint dislocation. Osteomyelitis is more common in the forefoot, is usually associated with a visible soft tissue tract (portal) on MRI, and rarely causes joint dislocation. Also, Charcot arthropathy frequently involves more than one bone and osteomyelitis is usually confined to one bone [14]. Referring the reader back to the algorithm, if the confirmatory test is negative for

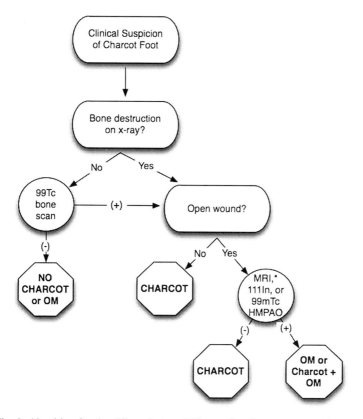

Fig. 5. Algorithm for the differentiation of Charcot foot from osteomyelitis (OM).

osteomyelitis, one has Charcot arthropathy. If it is positive, one has osteo-myelitis alone or osteomyelitis superimposed on Charcot arthropathy.

According to the algorithm, if no bone destruction is evident on plain ra-diograph, then a standard three-phase ^{99}Tc bone scan is sensitive to deter-mine if there is bone pathology. If the scan is negative, there is no Charcot foot and no osteomyelitis. If the scan is positive and there is no open wound, the diagnosis could be Charcot foot (while considering other diseases that result in a positive bone scan such as degenerative joint disease, rheumatoid arthritis, gout, fractures, and bone tumors) (Fig. 7A–C). If there is an open wound, follow the algorithm to "rule in" or "rule out" osteomy-elitis as described previously.

Classification and staging

Several authors have classified Charcot arthropathy by radiographic find-ings or anatomic location. The Eichenholtz Staging system is probably the

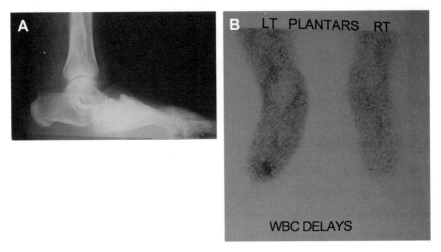

Fig. 6. (*A*) A lateral radiograph of the same patient as Fig. 2A, B showing equinus, tarsome-tatarsal subluxation, and a prominent cuboid plantarly. Note bone destruction evident on radiograph. (*B*) A white blood cell-labeled ^{99m}Tc HMPAO scan of the same patient as Fig. 6A revealing no increased uptake in the midfoot (cuboid), deep to the ulceration. The diagnosis is Charcot foot without osteomyelitis.

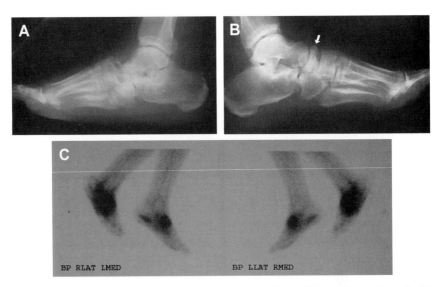

Fig. 7. (*A*) Lateral radiograph of the right foot in a male patient with bone destruction and mild deformity visible without clinical ulcerations. Note fragmentation and subluxation at the talo-navicular joint. (*B*) Lateral radiograph of the left foot in the same patient as Fig. 7A free of deformity but some resorptive changes are noted in the navicular (*arrow*). (*C*) A three-phase ^{99}Tc bone scan reveals increased activity in the midtarsal joints of both feet correlating with the radiographs in 7A and 7B. The diagnosis is Charcot foot without osteomyelitis.

most widely used and recognized. Shibata and colleagues [15] added an earlier, Stage 0, to the Eichenholtz classification, which describes warmth, dull pain, swelling, and joint instability in the midfoot of those with leprosy neuropathy, but normal-appearing joints on radiograph. Yu and Hudson [16] discussed the evaluation and treatment of Stage 0 Charcot foot in those with diabetic neuropathy and add the description of a fracture, sprain, or injury of the foot. Sella and Baratte [17] published a five-stage radiographic classification for medial-column neuropathic joint disease. They also describe a "pre-radiographic" clinical Stage 0. Sanders and Frykberg [18] classified Charcot arthropathy anatomically into patterns of joint involvement. Pattern I involves the forefoot joints, Pattern II involves the tarsometatarsal joint, Pattern III involves Chopart's joint or the naviculocuneiform joints, Pattern IV involves the ankle or subtalar joints, and Pattern V is isolated to the calcaneus.

While the previous classifications are useful in staging or describing the location of the joint involvement, they are not overtly prognostic. We propose a new classification that considers the complications associated with the Charcot joint, which may be a prognostic tool for amputation (Fig. 8). This is a two-axis system with the X-axis marking the anatomy affected including **1**. Forefoot; **2**. Midfoot; and **3**. Rearfoot/Ankle. The Y-axis

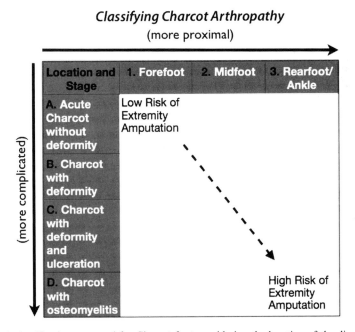

Fig. 8. A classification proposed for Charcot foot considering the location of the disease and the level of complexity. Note as one moves to the right and/or down the figure, we hypothesize that the risk of major amputation increases.

describes how complicated the Charcot joint is. **A** is acute Charcot with no deformity, **B** is Charcot foot with deformity, **C** is Charcot foot with deformity and ulceration, and **D** includes osteomyelitis. It makes clinical sense that as one moves across the X-axis or down the Y-axis the Charcot foot becomes "more complicated" and, thus, is at greater risk for amputation. Hence, we postulate that a 1A Charcot foot is relatively simple and at lower risk for amputation than a 3D Charcot foot. This new system combines the features of the clinical exam, radiography, and anatomy unlike the prior classifications.

Summary

Charcot arthropathy is a devastating progressive joint disease that is frequently disabling. Its diagnosis is often missed or delayed, resulting in more complications. A combination of clinical exam and imaging are necessary to correctly identify this disease as early as possible. Judicious use of three-phase ^{99}Tc bone scans is advocated, as they are nonspecific. They are not necessary when bone destruction is already evident on plain radiography. Osteomyelitis can be effectively differentiated from Charcot foot when following our simple algorithm. Additionally, when classifying Charcot joint disease, more consideration should be given to the complicating factors affecting the foot, such as deformity, ulceration, and osteomyelitis. The classification scheme we present in this article considers these factors and may help to prognosticate outcome.

References

[1] Pakarinen TK, Laine HJ, Honkonen SE, et al. Charcot arthropathy of the diabetic foot. Current concepts and review of 36 cases. Scand J Surg 2002;91(2):195–201.

[2] Chantelau E. The perils of procrastination: effects of early vs. delayed detection and treatment of incipient Charcot fracture. Diabet Med 2005;22(12):1707–12.

[3] Tan AL, Greenstein A, Jarrett SJ, et al. Acute neuropathic joint disease: a medical emergency? Diabetes Care 2005;28(12):2962–4.

[4] Foltz KD, Fallat LM, Schwartz S. Usefulness of a brief assessment battery for early detection of Charcot foot deformity in patients with diabetes. J Foot Ankle Surg 2004;43(2): 87–92.

[5] Stevens MJ, Edmonds ME, Foster AV, et al. Selective neuropathy and preserved vascular responses in the diabetic Charcot foot. Diabetologia 1992;35(2):148–54.

[6] Lavery LA, Higgins KR, Holguin D, et al. Home skin temperature monitoring reduces the incidence of diabetic foot complications. Diabetes 2002;51(Suppl 1):1039.

[7] Foto JG, Brasseaux D, Birke JA. Essential features of a handheld infrared thermometer used to guide the treatment of neuropathic feet. J Am Podiatr Med Assoc 2007;97(5):360–5.

[8] Armstrong DG, Lavery LA. Monitoring healing of acute Charcot's arthropathy with infrared dermal thermometry. J Rehabil Res Dev 1997;34:317–21.

[9] Eichenholtz SN. Charcot joints. Springfield (IL): Charles C. Thomas; 1966.

[10] Schauwecker DS, Park HM, Mock BH, et al. Evaluation of complicating osteomyelitis with Tc-99m MDP, In-111 granulocytes, and Ga-67 citrate. J Nucl Med 1984;25(8):849–53.

[11] Poirier JY, Garin E, Derrien C, et al. Diagnosis of osteomyelitis in the diabetic foot with a 99mTc-HMPAO leucocyte scintigraphy combined with a 99mTc-MDP bone scintigraphy. Diabetes Metab 2002;28(6 Pt 1):485–90.

[12] Ledermann HP, Morrison WB. Differential diagnosis of pedal osteomyelitis and diabetic neuroarthropathy: MR imaging. Semin Musculoskelet Radiol 2005;9(3):272–83.

[13] Seabold JE, Flickinger FW, Kao SC, et al. Indium-111-leukocyte/technetium-99m-MDP bone and magnetic resonance imaging: difficulty of diagnosing osteomyelitis in patients with neuropathic osteoarthropathy. J Nucl Med 1990;31(5):549–56.

[14] Morrison WB, Schweitzer ME, Batte WG, et al. Osteomyelitis of the foot: relative importance of primary and secondary MR imaging signs. Radiology 1998;207(3):625–32.

[15] Shibata T, Tada K, Hashizume C. The results of arthrodesis of the ankle for leprotic neuroarthropathy. J Bone Joint Surg Am 1990;72:749–56.

[16] Yu GV, Hudson JR. Evaluation and treatment of stage 0 Charcot's neuroarthropathy of the foot and ankle. J Am Podiatr Med Assoc 2002;92(4):210–20.

[17] Sella EJ, Barrette C. Staging of Charcot neuroarthropathy along the medial column of the foot in the diabetic patient. J Foot Ankle Surg 1999;38(1):34–40.

[18] Sanders LJ, Frykberg RG. The Charcot foot. In: Frykberg, editor. The high risk foot in diabetes mellitus. New York: Churchill Livingstone; 1991. p. 325–35.

ELSEVIER
SAUNDERS

Clin Podiatr Med Surg
25 (2008) 53–62

CLINICS IN
PODIATRIC
MEDICINE AND
SURGERY

The Natural History of Charcot's Neuroarthropathy

David L. Nielson, DPM[a],*,
David G. Armstrong, DPM, PhD[b]

[a]Center for Lower Extremity Ambulatory Research, Dr. William M. Scholl
College of Podiatric Medicine at Rosalind Franklin University of Medicine and Science,
3333 Green Bay Road, North Chicago, IL 60064, USA
[b]Dr. William M. Scholl College of Podiatric Medicine at Rosalind Franklin University
of Medicine and Science, 3333 Green Bay Road, North Chicago, IL 60064, USA

In the autumn of 1827, John Kearsley Mitchell [1] (1798–1858) of Phila-delphia described a patient as "affected with caries of the spine, was suddenly attacked with all the usual symptoms of acute rheumatism of the lower extremities. One ankle, and the knee of the opposite leg, tumefied, red, hot and painful..." "The usual treatment by leeches, purgatives, and...evaporating lotions, had the effect of transferring the symptoms to the other ankle and knee...disappointed in the treatment, I began to suspect that the cause of the irritation might lie in the affected spine..."

Silas Weir Mitchell (1829–1914), an experimental physiologist and neurologist during the American Civil War, saw injuries related to the nerves and coined the term *causalgia*. Mitchell and colleagues [2] described alterations in the nutrition of joints, "We have ourselves seen cases of spinal injury, in which rheumatic symptoms seemed to have been among the consequences...The indisputable fact (is) that there are rheumatisms depending for existence on neural changes..."

l'Hospice de la Salpêtrière Paris, the largest charitable hospital in Europe in 1862 with approximately 5000 residents, was also known as the "grand asylum of human misery" and "museum of living pathology." Jean-Marie Charcot transformed the Salpêtrière into a great teaching and research center for diseases of the nervous system. Charcot [3] describes a method that included extensive clinical observation, detailed notes, documentation of changes in status, anatomic drawings, and microscopic depictions. Signs

---

* Corresponding author.
E-mail address: david.l.nielson@gmail.com (D.L. Nielson).

0891-8422/08/$ - see front matter. Published by Elsevier Inc.
doi:10.1016/j.cpm.2007.10.004

were correlated with symptoms and anatomic changes. Sanders and Hoche [4] translated his writings into English.

At the Seventh International Medical Conference, James Paget declared, "This disease is, in fact, a distinct pathological entity, and deserves the name, by which it will be known as 'Charcot's disease'" [5]. In 1936, William Riely Jordan [6] associated neuropathy as a complication of diabetes mellitus. More historical information has since become available and is beautifully reviewed at the beginning of this issue (see the article by Sanders elsewhere in this issue).

Before the advent of insulin in the 1920s, neuroarthropathy was not seen in patients who had diabetes but was certainly associated with other diseases, especially tabes dorsalis. Box 1 lists the common causes of Charcot's neuroarthropathy.

As a result of the dramatically increased life span yielded by widespread insulin use, many complications of diabetes—not the least of which is Charcot's neuroarthropathy—became widely evident and are now almost exclusive to this disease [7]. Studies vary in the incidence of Charcot's neuroarthropathy in the diabetic patient who has neuropathy. Lavery and colleagues [8] reported that in a study of 1666 patients followed up for 24 months, the incidence of Charcot's neuroarthropathy was 8.5 per 1000 per year.

Lack of perception of 4 or more of 10 sites on the bottom of the foot using the Semmes-Weinstein monofilament (SWMF), carries 97% sensitivity and 83% specificity in identifying patients at highest risk for diabetic foot ulcers. This was the optimum combination of sensitivity and specificity for this device. Another device commonly used in diabetic foot specialty clinics, the biothesiometer, measures vibration perception, also known as vibratory perception threshold (VPT). The optimum VPT was 25 V, yielding 90% sensitivity and 84% specificity in detecting neuropathy. When these diagnostic modalities were combined (with one or both positive on physical examination), the sensitivity rose to 100%, with a specificity of 77%. Clearly, a combination of modalities leads to a more sensitive (and not significantly less specific) screening tool [9].

Box 1. Common causes of Charcot's neuroarthropathy

Syphilis
Tabes dorsalis
Leprosy
Syringomyelia
Spina bifida
Meningomyelocele
Chronic alcoholism
Spinal injury
Diabetes

Many theories exist for the cause and pathophysiology of Charcot's disease of the joint, which are described in detail in another article in this issue (see the article by Jeffcoate and colleagues elsewhere in this issue). The German theory is indirectly supported by a study that identified increased pressures to the foot with added glycosylation of the Achilles tendon, creating added pressure on the forefoot, which causes a collapse in the midfoot. This collapse is located at the tarsometatarsal and talonavicular/calcaneal cuboid joints, which is the most common site for acute Charcot's neuroarthropathy foot deformities [10–12].

Registered at the Foot Ulcers Trial Unit, were anonymized details on more than 200 cases of acute Charcot's neuroarthropathy (April 2005–December 2006) that document demographic details, possible triggers, complications, treatments, and outcomes. Jeffcoate and colleagues [13] and other investigators [14–18] are evaluating the potential role of cytokines, specifically receptor activator for nuclear factor-κB ligand (RANK-L) and osteoprotegerin (OPG), and suggest that an imbalance in these cytokines may be responsible for the inflammatory effects on the degeneration of bone.

Clinical manifestations of Charcot's arthropathy process

A common mechanical manifestation of Charcot's arthropathy occurs when a functionally shorter Achilles tendon leads to an equinus deformity. This causes increased pressure in the forefoot. When coupled with fulminant inflammation and weakened ligamentous support, breakdown may and often does occur at the midfoot (Fig. 1). The biomechanics of the foot are now in an abnormal position, with increased pressures causing further deformity of an unstable foot type.

Dyck and colleagues [19] describe that as glucose levels increase, the lumen of the blood vessels enlarge. This, in turn, decreases the ability of blood to carry oxygen and nutrients across the wall to the surrounding tissue, especially the nerves. Because the nerve is deprived of oxygen and nutrients, nerve damage ensues. These investigators argue this to be the underlying cause of neuropathy.

Before 1997, there were no studies in the literature to describe the clinical characteristics and treatment course of acute Charcot's arthropathy. In a prospective study, Armstrong and colleagues [11] found that the mean time for immobilization of the foot affected by Charcot's arthropathy was 6 months. During this time, skin temperatures, edema, and radiographic appearance normalized.

The joint affected by Charcot's arthropathy is a joint that lacks the ability to respond by means of reflexes to abnormal stresses. As a consequence, the subchondral bone of the involved joint disintegrates, leading to joint collapse and, usually, considerable joint deformity. As the underlying disease process worsens, the gait pattern becomes increasingly ataxic, leading to

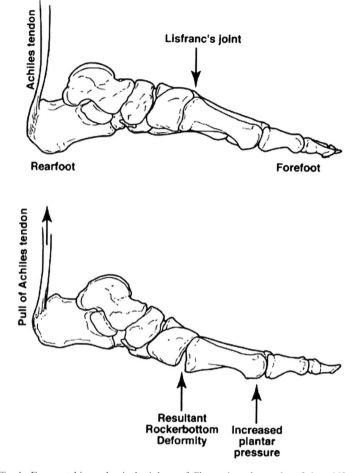

Fig. 1. Frequent biomechanical etiology of Charcot's arthropathy of the midfoot.

increasing stress on the lower extremity joints. Subsequent large fracture formations are a major factor in initiating the considerable joint changes.

The pathogenesis of the joint affected by Charcot's arthropathy may be defined as a "vicious cycle" of injury and repair. After initial injury, the inflammatory phase initiates an increase in localized blood flow, along with increased histiocytic and osteoclastic activity, removal of blood clots, and resorption of the avascular bone. In the following repair phase, new bone is laid down, producing callus around the fracture sites. Unfortunately, this normal cycle of healing is relatively inefficient, because the bone resorption, which occurred during the inflammatory phase, leaves the resultant atrophic bone easily traumatized even after walking, and the process starts again.

The joints most frequently affected by the pathologic changes of Charcot's arthropathy are the weight-bearing joints, predominantly the midfoot but also the hind foot, ankle, knees, and hips. The reported distribution within the diabetic neuropathic foot is 60% at the tarsal and metatarsal joints, 30% at the metatarsophalangeal joints, and 10% at the ankle [20,21]. When the mid-foot/midtarsal region is affected, the deformity may result in a prolapsed arch, producing a rocker-bottom foot or a valgus or varus deviation of the forefoot. With a collapsed arch, mechanical stresses are supported during midstance, leading to progressive degeneration of osseous structures and the underlying skin. Consequently, ulcer formation, deep infection, and increased bone destruction are possible outcomes. Severe valgus or varus deformity of the foot and ankle results in large gait forces directed to small areas, such as the malleoli, that are not designed to support.

Charcot's disease of the joint can present in two different ways when viewed radiographically: atrophic and hypertrophic. Atrophic patterns have characteristic dissolution of bone and joint surfaces, commonly seen in the lesser metatarsal regions. The hypertrophic pattern is more common and can present anywhere within the foot. The pattern can be divided into three stages:

1. Fragmentation: the active phase of Charcot's disease; this involves destruction, whereby bony fragmentation and joint disruption are visible, leaving osseous debris surrounding the affected joint.
2. Coalescence: healing phase, whereby the osseous debris is resorbed and new bone is laid down. Patterns of trabeculation may be seen across the fractured margins on radiographs.
3. Reconstruction: remodeling phase, which can last from several months to years. Bone integrity is strengthened, and joints are re-established in the form of pseudoarthroses or fusions. The progression of healing during the reconstruction phase determines the outcome of the joints involved. Generally, forefoot and midfoot involvement respond favorably, whereas rearfoot and ankle involvement is more complicated

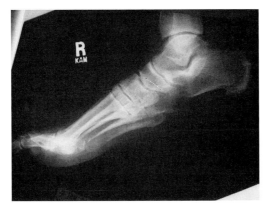

Fig. 2. Initial radiographic presentation of acute early-stage Charcot's arthropathy.

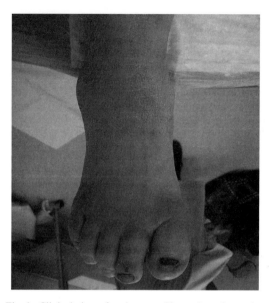

Fig. 3. Clinical view of early-stage Charcot's arthropathy.

with a poorer prognosis. This is attributable to the severe destruction of ligamentous structures that previously offered a large proportion of support and joint integrity in these areas. It should be noted that some investigators have added a "stage 0," which is described as acute injury without radiographic evidence [22,23].

In earlier studies into the pathologic findings of joints affected with Charcot's arthropathy, it was suggested that the initial changes occurred in the joint cartilage and subchondral bone rather than in the bone itself.

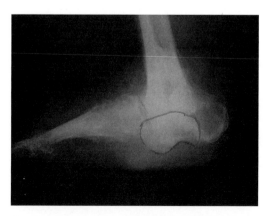

Fig. 4. Late-stage chronic Charcot's arthropathy. Radiograph shows bony and ligamentous positional changes in a patient who has long-standing untreated Charcot's arthropathy.

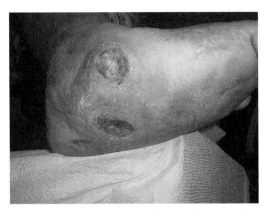

Fig. 5. Same patient with ulceration secondary to increased pressure from midfoot collapse.

These changes are triggered by a series of reactive events producing inflammatory changes in the synovium and capsule. Inflammation of the joint complex allows the lax joint to be easily subluxed and traumatized, particularly when proprioception is diminished, creating damage to the joint surface and underlying bone. Consequent complications include osteophytic growths, cartilage erosion, chip and compression fractures, intraarticular and extra-articular exostosis, and ossification of the ligamentous structures. Because neuropathy is present, the changes are often undetected by the individual until the joint is totally destroyed or there is skin breakdown with possible infection. Several factors contribute to the pathogenesis of joints affected with Charcot's arthropathy. These include continual trauma (repetitive microtrauma or an isolated major trauma) and neurologic conditions (diminished pain sensation and proprioception) [24].

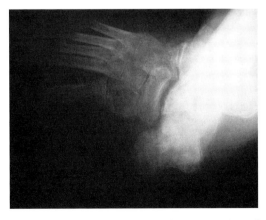

Fig. 6. Clear dislocation at the talonavicular joint. The talus is plantarflexed and medially dislocated.

Initial stages of acute Charcot's arthropathy

Treatment goals in the acute phase are to avoid fracture, dislocations, instability, and deformity, thereby obtaining a stable minimally deformed foot (Figs. 2–6). Bisphosphonates slow the activity of osteoclastic absorption of bone, which slows the rate of the Charcot's arthropathy process [25–27]. Focusing on a different path, the imbalance of RANK-L and OPG may be addressed through the use of currently available agents, such as salmon calcitonin [28], and perhaps with such agents as tumor necrosis factor-α (TNFα) inhibitors or anticancer therapeutics with RANK-L inhibition properties, such as sulforaphane [29].

Uncontrolled diabetes and even the long-term effects of controlled diabetes can be devastating. Early diagnosis and start of treatment are crucial as steps in prevention, or further progression of the disease may occur. Glycemic

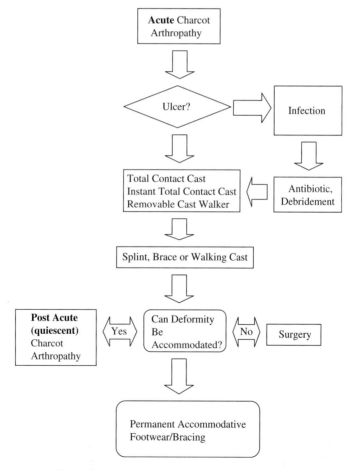

Fig. 7. Treatment algorithm of Charcot's arthropathy.

control [30] and offloading [31] may be important in the mitigation or prevention of further morphologic changes in the foot. Once the foot becomes stable (ie, after contact casting or a similar aggressive method of immobilization), a more long-term method of protection may be used (ie, depth inlay versus molded shoes, Charcot restraint orthotic walkers, bracing) (Fig. 7).

Charcot's neuroarthropathy is one of the most debilitating progressive diseases. Charcot's neuroarthropathy is often mistaken for gout, fractures, or infection. Patients who have diabetes and neuropathy and present with a hot, swollen, erythematous foot should, in many cases, carry a diagnosis of Charcot's neuroarthropathy until proven otherwise. A high index of suspicion, coupled with aggressive intervention and protection, is likely the optimal combination to prevent the often deleterious consequences of this malady.

References

[1] Mitchell JK. On a new practice in acute and chronic rheumatism. Am J Med Sci 1831;8:55–64.
[2] Mitchell SW, Morehouse GR, Keen WW. Gunshot wounds and other injuries of nerves. 1864. Clin Orthop Relat Res 2007 May;458:35–9.
[3] Charcot JM. Sur quelques arthropathies qui paraissent dependre d'une lesion du cerveau ou de la moelle epiniere. Arch Physiol Norm Path 1868;1:161–71.
[4] Charcot JM. On some arthopathics apparently related to a lesion of the brain or spinal cord. In: Sanders L, Hoche G, editors. Journal of the history of the neurosciences (translated and edited) 1992;1:75–87.
[5] MacCormac W. Transactions of the International Medical Congress: seventh session held in London, August 2–9, 1881. vol. 1. p. 128–9.
[6] Jordan WR. Neuritic manifestations in diabetes mellitus. Arch Intern Med 1936;57:307–12.
[7] Harris MI, Eastman R, Cowle C. Symptoms of sensory neuropathy in adults with NIDDM in the US population. Diabetes Care 1993;16:446–52.
[8] Lavery LA, Armstrong DG, Wunderlich RP, et al. Diabetic foot syndrome. Diabetes Care 2003;26:1435–8.
[9] Armstrong DG, Lavery LA, Vela SA, et al. Choosing a practical screening instrument to identify patients at risk for diabetic foot ulceration. Arch Intern Med 1998;148:289–92.
[10] Armstrong DG, Lavery LA. Elevated peak plantar pressures in patients who have Charcot arthropathy. J Bone Joint Surg Am 1998;80(3):365 9.
[11] Armstrong DG, Todd WF, Lavery LA, et al. The natural history of acute Charcot's arthropathy in a diabetic foot specialty clinic. Diabet Med 1997;14:357–63.
[12] Cavanagh PR, Young MJ, Adams JE, et al. Radiographic abnormalities in the feet of patients with diabetic neuropathy. Diabetes Care 1994;17:201–9.
[13] Catlow R, Jeffcoate W, Baker N, et al. Diabetic foot ulcer trial. Available at: www.charcot.org.uk. Accessed August 2, 2007.
[14] Jeffcoate W, Game F, Cavanagh PR. The role of proinflammatory cytokines in the cause of neuropathic osteoarthropathy (acute Charcot foot) in diabetes. Lancet 2005;366:2058–61.
[15] Cappellen D, Luong-Nguyen NH, Bongiovanni S, et al. Transcriptional program of mouse osteoclast differentiation governed by the macrophage colony-stimulating factor and the ligand for the receptor activator of NF-kappaB. J Biol Chem 2002;277(24):21971–82.
[16] Anand DV, Lahiri A, Lim E, et al. The relationship between plasma osteoprotegerin levels and coronary artery calcification in uncomplicated type 2 diabetic subjects. J Am Coll Cardiol 2006;47:1850–7.

[17] Grimaud E, Soubigou L, Couillaud S, et al. Receptor activator of nuclear factor-κB ligand (RANKL)/osteoprotegerin (OPG) ratio is increased in severe randomized. Am J Pathol 2003;163:2021–31.

[18] Pettit AR, Walsh NC, Manning C, et al. RANKL protein is expressed at the pannus-bone interface at sites of articular bone erosion in rheumatoid arthritis. Rheumatology 2006; 45(9):1068–76.

[19] Dyck PJ, Zimmerman BR, Vilen TH, et al. Nerve glucose, fructose, sorbitol, myo-inositol, and fiber degeneration and regeneration in diabetic neuropathy. N Engl J Med 1988;319: 542–8.

[20] Harrelson JM. Management of the diabetic foot. The Orthopaedic Clinics of North America 1989;(99):605–19.

[21] Schon LC, Weinfeld SB, Horton GA, et al. Radiographic and clinical classification of acquired midtarsus deformities. Foot Ankle Int 1998;19(6):394–404.

[22] Yu GV, Hudson JR. Evaluation and treatment of stage 0 Charcot's neuroarthropathy of the foot and ankle. J Am Podiatr Med Assoc 2002;92(4):210–20.

[23] Sella EJ, Barrette C. Staging of Charcot neuroarthropathy along the medial column of the foot in the diabetic patient. J Foot Ankle Surg 1999;38(1):34–40.

[24] Sanders LJ, Frykberg RG. Charcot neuroarthropathy of the foot. In: Bowker JH, Pfeifer MA, editors. Levin and O'Neal's the diabetic foot. 6th edition. Saint Louis (Missouri): Mosby; 2001. p. 439–62.

[25] Jude EB, Selby PL, Boulton AJ. Bisphosphonates in the treatment of Charcot neuroarthropathy: a double-blind randomized controlled trial. Diabetologia 2001;44:2032–7.

[26] Anderson JJ, Woelffer KE, Holtzman JJ, et al. Bisphosphonates for the treatment of Charcot neuroarthropathy. J Foot Ankle Surg 2004;285–9.

[27] Childs M, Armstrong DG, Edelson GW. Is Charcot arthropathy a late sequela of osteoporosis in patients with diabetes mellitus? J Foot Ankle Surg 1998;37:437–9.

[28] Bem R, Jirkovská A, Fejfarová V, et al. Intranasal calcitonin in the treatment of acute Charcot neuro-osteoarthropathy: a randomized controlled trial. Diabetes Care 2006;29(6): 1392–4.

[29] Kim SJ, Kang SY, Shin HH, et al. Sulforaphane inhibits osteoclastogenesis by inhibiting nuclear factor-kappaB. Mol Cells 2005;20(3):364–70.

[30] Tesfaye S, Stevens LK, Stephenson JM, et al. Prevalence of diabetic peripheral neuropathy and its relation to glycaemic control and potential risk factors: the EURODIAB IDDM complication study. Diabetologia 1996;39:1377–84.

[31] Armstrong DG, Lavery LA. Evidence-based options for offloading diabetic wounds. Clin Podiatr Med Surg 1998;15(1):95–103.

ELSEVIER
SAUNDERS

Clin Podiatr Med Surg
25 (2008) 63–69

CLINICS IN
PODIATRIC
MEDICINE AND
SURGERY

Medical Treatment of Charcot Neuroosteoarthropathy

Andreas Jostel, MD, Edward B. Jude, MD, MRCP*

*Tameside Acute NHS Trust, Fountain Street, Ashton-under-Lyne,
Lancashire, OL6 9RW, UK*

The pathophysiology of Charcot neuroosteoarthropathy (CN) is still incompletely understood, although main etiological components have been identified [1,2], and recent insights into the molecular mechanisms of resorptive bone diseases have revealed promising candidate targets of new medical therapy [3,4].

The sine qua non of CN is the presence of severe peripheral neuropathy, most commonly seen in patients with diabetes mellitus. Trauma (sometimes very subtle and possibly unnoticed by the patient) is widely believed to be the essential triggering factor for the development of CN. Hyperemia of the affected foot is an important cofactor, and may be the consequence of sympathetic denervation in autonomic neuropathy or of an abnormal sympathetic response to injury similar to reflex sympathetic dystrophy. The bones involved in CN are typically osteopenic even before the development of CN, and this is likely to play a role in facilitating the development of microfractures as an initiating event [5–7].

Early acute CN is characterized by edema, erythema, warmth, and typically mild to moderate pain and tenderness (despite the presence of neuropathy)—classical signs of an acute inflammatory process, which explains the potential for confusion with conditions such as cellulitis, deep vein thrombosis, other arthropathies, or osteomyelitis (in the presence of a concomitant diabetic foot ulcer). Misdiagnosis and delay of immediate treatment (offloading and immobilization) allow the perpetuation of mechanical stress and microtrauma, leading to fracture-dislocation, bone fragmentation, and resorption, resulting in joint disorganization and ultimately irreversible joint deformity with significant disability and high risk of complications [8,9]. Even with rapid recognition and immediate offloading, quiescence of the condition is often

---

* Corresponding author.
E-mail address: edward.jude@tgh.nhs.uk (E.B. Jude).

0891-8422/08/$ - see front matter © 2008 Elsevier Inc. All rights reserved.
doi:10.1016/j.cpm.2007.09.001
podiatric.theclinics.com

only achieved after several months of joint immobilization, suggesting a prolonged activation of the disease process at the cellular level, which has become the main focus of adjuvant medical therapy of CN.

Nonpharmacological therapy

Elimination of physical stress to the Charcot joint ("offloading") is essential to break the vicious cycle of repeated trauma propagating the acute phase of CN. Offloading remains the cornerstone of therapy even with adjunctive pharmacological treatments, and is best achieved with a total contact cast (TCC) and reduction of weight bearing, resulting in improvement of clinical markers within 2 weeks of application [10]. Average use of a cast is approximately 12 to 18 weeks, and healing time is significantly reduced with early institution of treatment and proper adherence to partial weight-bearing instructions [11,12]. Alternatives to the TCC such as removable cast walkers have the benefit of being instantly applicable without specialist skills, but compliance with a removable device is significantly reduced [13], and making the cast irremovable with additional bands of plaster has been advocated ("instant total-contact cast") [14].

Increased osteoclastic activity as target of pharmacological therapy

Radiographs of Charcot joints typically demonstrate evidence of concomitant avid bone resorption and apposition, suggesting high local bone turnover rates. Studies of various bone turnover markers have confirmed these abnormalities in bone metabolism in acute CN.

Edelson and colleagues [15] found increased urinary levels of cross-linked N-telopeptides of type 1 collagen (NTX), confirming increased levels of collagen breakdown in subjects with CN. Gough and colleagues [16] demonstrated increased serum levels of pyridinoline cross-linked carboxy-terminal telopeptide domain of type 1 collagen (1CTP) but unchanged levels of carboxy-terminal propeptide of type 1 collagen (P1CP) in diabetic patients with acute CN, indicative of increased bone turnover not matched by an increase in bone formation.

In a study by Selby and colleagues [17], patients with acute CN had increased levels of both urinary deoxypyridinoline and bone-specific alkaline phosphatase, suggesting increased activity of bone resorption as well as bone formation, ie, an ongoing remodeling process. These biochemical findings are similar to other conditions with excessive bone turnover, such as Paget's disease of the bone, hypercalcemia of malignancy, and osteoporosis.

Bisphosphonates

Pharmacological agents able to inhibit pathological bone resorption are logical treatment options for diseases associated with excessive bone turnover. The most common therapy to date is use of bisphosphonates (BP), which were first synthesized in 1865 and have been used in medicine since 1968 [18], mainly for their antiresorptive properties in conditions with increased bone turnover. BP are stable pyrophosphate analogs, in which the oxygen atom of the pyrophosphate molecule P-O-P is replaced by a carbon atom (P-C-P), making it resistant to enzymatic hydrolysis. First-generation BP have non–nitrogen-containing carbon side chains (etidronate, clodronate), whereas second-generation BP (alendronate, pamidronate, zoledronic acid) carry nitrogen-containing side chains. The carbon side chains determine the pharmacological properties of the BP, giving exponentially increased antiresorptive potency in comparison to etidronate for the more potent bisphosphonates clodronate (factor 10), pamidronate, alendronate, ibandronate/risedronate, and zoledronate (factor > 10,000) [18]. The effect on cell metabolism after internalization by osteoclasts varies between first- and second-generation bisphosphonates: non–nitrogen-containing first-generation bisphosphonates (etidronate, clodronate) are metabolized to cytotoxic ATP analogs, inducing osteoclast apoptosis [19]. Nitrogen-containing bisphosphonates (including pamidronate, alendronate, ibandronate, risedronate, zoledronic acid) inhibit farnesyl diphosphonate (FPP) synthase in the biosynthetic mevalonate pathway, interfering with the synthesis of signaling molecules affecting cell structure and function and survival of osteoclasts [20]. They may also have a weak inhibitory effect on osteoblast apoptosis.

An open-labeled pilot study by Selby and colleagues [21] investigated the effects of bisphosphonate treatment in six patients with active CN by administering a total of six pamidronate infusions over a period of 10 weeks (60 mg at first visit, then 30 mg every 2 weeks). Patients' symptoms improved, and a significant fall in foot temperature by 2.4°C was recorded. Alkaline phosphatase levels as markers of bone turnover decreased significantly by 25%.

The preliminary data of that study prompted a larger, randomized placebo-controlled double-blind trial by Jude and colleagues [10]. Thirty-nine type 2 diabetic patients with active CN were recruited from four centers in the United Kingdom, and received a single infusion of either 90 mg Pamidronate or normal saline (placebo) at baseline in addition to standard care of foot immobilization (with Scotch cast boot, pneumatic walker, or TCC) and bed rest. Clinical and biochemical markers of disease activity were measured over the 12-month study period.

Foot temperatures (as measured with an infrared thermometer at the site of maximum deformity and compared with the contralateral foot) fell significantly in both groups at 2 weeks, with a further fall at 4 weeks in the treatment group only, which did not reach statistical significance in comparison with the placebo group. Patients' symptom scores (measured with visual analog scales every 3 months) improved significantly more in the treatment group compared with the placebo group for all posttreatment assessments.

Bone resorption markers (second-void early morning urinary deoxypyri-dinoline, measured as ratio to urinary creatinine; and serum bone-specific alkaline phosphatase) were measured during the study. Deoxypyridininoline was significantly decreased in the treatment group at 2 to 6 weeks, with a gradual return to baseline values in the following 18 weeks. Bone-specific alkaline phosphatase levels followed a similar pattern: it was significantly reduced from 4 to 12 weeks, with a gradual return to baseline over the subsequent 40 weeks.

In a study by Anderson and colleagues [22], the short-term effects of pamidronate infusion of variable dose on acute CN were evaluated retrospectively in 13 patients and compared with 10 control patients who did not receive bisphosphonate treatment. A statistically significantly greater reduction in temperature was seen in the treatment group at 2 days and 2 weeks, and alkaline phosphatase levels decreased significantly more in the treatment group at 2 weeks. A common side effect of a drug-induced fever was noted in 6 of 10 treatment patients, which lasted no more than 24 hours in any of the patients.

In another study by Pitocco and colleagues [23], oral alendronate (70 mg weekly) was used in a randomized controlled trial in 11 patients compared with placebo in 9 control patients with acute CN. Study assessments took place at baseline and again at 6 months. A significantly greater reduction in foot temperature was seen in the treatment group at 6 months. Pain scores on a visual analog scale improved significantly only in the treatment group at the follow-up assessment. Serum collagen COOH-terminal telopeptide of type 1 collagen (1CTP), and hydroxyprolin decreased significantly in the treatment group after 6 months, and a similar trend was seen in alkaline phosphatase levels. Bone mineral density assessed by dual-energy x-ray absorptiometry demonstrated significantly improved mineralization for the total foot and distal phalanges in the bisphosphonate group.

Other antiresorptive agents

Calcitonin is a 32–amino acid peptide synthesized in thyroid medullary cells that has a direct inhibitory effect on osteoclasts via calcitonin receptors. Osteoclast responsiveness to calcitonin varies greatly among species, and the physiological role in humans is still not fully understood [19]. Long-term administration of supraphysiological doses (or the much more potent salmon calcitonin) is known to result in receptor down-regulation and an escape phenomenon. The main effect of calcitonin on osteoclast activity appears to be exerted via inhibition of cytoplasmic motility, secretory activity, and a reduction in the number of osteoclasts [24].

Calcitonin has been used to a lesser extent than bisphosphonates for treatment of osteoporosis, partly because of the need for parenteral administration (subcutaneously or nasally). Long-term administration of the most commonly used preparation of salmon calcitonin is known to cause calcitonin receptor down-regulation, causing an escape phenomenon, and there is a potential for antibody formation. Advantages over bisphosphonates are possible stimulation of bone formation and its use irrespective of renal insufficiency.

Bem and colleagues [25] performed a randomized controlled trial of intranasal calcitonin (200 IU daily) and oral calcium versus oral calcium alone in 32 diabetic patients with acute CN in addition to standard care of CN. The trial also included five patients with renal insufficiency. Treatment with calcitonin was associated with significantly greater reduction in 1CTP levels during the first 3 months; bone-specific alkaline phosphatase levels were significantly decreased at 3 months compared with the control group. Foot skin temperature reduced irrespective of calcitonin treatment. The findings applied to both patients with normal and abnormal renal functions.

Proinflammatory cytokine pathways as targets of medical therapy

The presenting clinical features of an acute Charcot joint suggest a significant inflammatory component as part of the disease process. Recent research has elucidated molecular pathways by which an exaggerated inflammatory response contributes to excessive osteoclast activation in CN, which promises attractive medical treatment options in the future.

The discovery of osteoprotegerin (OPG) as a molecule that causes profound decrease in osteoclast numbers and osteopetrosis was a major scientific discovery in bone biology in 1997 [26]. This was followed by the identification of RANKL as its natural ligand, and RANK as its sole receptor on osteoclast progenitor cells, responsible for the transformation into mature osteoclasts [27]. Numerous cytokines and hormones have since been identified to act via the osteoblast by modulating the OPG/RANK balance, thereby regulating osteoclast formation [19]. Stimulants of osteoclastogenesis include interleukin (IL)-1, IL-6, tumor necrosis factor (TNF)-alpha, parathyroid hormone, and 1,12(OH)2D3; inhibitors include IL-4, transforming growth factor (TGF)-beta, interferon gamma, and calcitonin.

A hypothesis that links the inflammatory component of acute CN to the abnormalities in bone metabolism is based on these pathways [3]. An initial bone fracture or microtrauma may trigger an exaggerated inflammatory response in an insensate, hyperemic foot, with the excessive release of proinflammatory cytokines, such as TNF-alpha and IL-1beta. These proinflammatory cytokines stimulate overexpression of RANKL, which in turn leads to maturation of osteoclasts, leading to the typical osteolysis of CN. Overexpression of TNF-alpha, IL-1, and IL-6 have indeed been demonstrated at increased levels in pathological specimens of CN [4].

It is therefore plausible that TNF-alpha antagonists as well as high-dose corticosteroids (which decrease nuclear factor [NF]-kappaB expression) may have a beneficial role in the treatment of acute CN, but clinical experience is as yet lacking. Future medical anti-inflammatory therapy may also include inhibitors of RANKL, NF-kappaB, and IL-1beta, which have been used in animal studies to attenuate inflammatory arthritis.

Summary

    The cornerstone of treatment of acute CN is immediate effective offloading, typically with total contact casting, and reduction in weight bearing. The main current targets of pharmacological intervention are the inhibition of excess osteoclast activation and suppression of an excess proinflammatory cytokine response. Antiresorptive therapy, especially with bisphosphonates, has been used in randomized trials. While evidence of an ideal dosage regime and significant differences in long-term outcome are lacking and should be evaluated in future studies, the trials so far demonstrated improved symptom control, a more rapid decline in foot temperature, and a significant decrease in bone turnover markers, with no demonstration of significant harmful effects. Growing insight into molecular pathways of resorptive bone disease will undoubtedly facilitate novel adjunctive pharmacological therapies.

References

[1] Hartemann-Heurtier A, Van GH, Grimaldi A. The Charcot foot. Lancet 2002;360(9347): 1776–9.
[2] Boulton AJ. The diabetic foot: from art to science. The 18th Camillo Golgi lecture. Diabetologia 2004;47(8):1343–53.
[3] Jeffcoate WJ, Game F, Cavanagh PR. The role of proinflammatory cytokines in the cause of neuropathic osteoarthropathy (acute Charcot foot) in diabetes. Lancet 2005;366(9502): 2058–61.
[4] Baumhauer JF, O'Keefe RJ, Schon LC, et al. Cytokine-induced osteoclastic bone resorption in Charcot arthropathy: an immunohistochemical study. Foot Ankle Int 2006;27(10): 797–800.
[5] Young MJ, Marshall A, Adams JE, et al. Osteopenia, neurological dysfunction, and the development of Charcot neuroarthropathy. Diabetes Care 1995;18(1):34–8.
[6] Larsen K, Fabrin J, Holstein PE. Incidence and management of ulcers in diabetic Charcot feet. J Wound Care 2001;10(8):323–8.
[7] Herbst SA, Jones KB, Saltzman CL. Pattern of diabetic neuropathic arthropathy associated with the peripheral bone mineral density. J Bone Joint Surg Br 2004;86(3):378–83.
[8] Tan AL, Greenstein A, Jarrett SJ, et al. Acute neuropathic joint disease: a medical emergency? Diabetes Care 2005;28(12):2962–4.
[9] Chantelau E. The perils of procrastination: effects of early vs. delayed detection and treatment of incipient Charcot fracture. Diabet Med 2005;22(12):1707–12.
[10] Jude EB, Selby PL, Burgess J, et al. Bisphosphonates in the treatment of Charcot neuroarthropathy: a double-blind randomised controlled trial. Diabetologia 2001;44(11):2032–7.
[11] Sinacore DR. Acute Charcot arthropathy in patients with diabetes mellitus: healing times by foot location. J Diabetes Complications 1998;12(5):287–93.
[12] Armstrong DG, Todd WF, Lavery LA, et al. The natural history of acute Charcot's arthropathy in a diabetic foot specialty clinic. Diabet Med 1997;14(5):357–63.
[13] Armstrong DG, Lavery LA, Kimbriel HR, et al. Activity patterns of patients with diabetic foot ulceration: patients with active ulceration may not adhere to a standard pressure offloading regimen. Diabetes Care 2003;26(9):2595–7.

[14] Armstrong DG, Short B, Espensen EH, et al. Technique for fabrication of an "instant total-contact cast" for treatment of neuropathic diabetic foot ulcers. J Am Podiatr Med Assoc 2002;92(7):405–8.

[15] Edelson GW, Jensen JL, Kaczynski R. Identifying acute Charcot arthropathy through urinarycross-linked N-telopeptides. Diabetes 1996;45(Suppl 2):108A.

[16] Gough A, Abraha H, Li F, et al. Measurement of markers of osteoclast and osteoblast activity in patients with acute and chronic diabetic Charcot neuroarthropathy. Diabet Med 1997;14(7):527–31.

[17] Selby PL, Jude EB, Burgess J, et al. Bone turnover markers in acute Charcot neuroarthropathy. Diabetologia 1998;41(Suppl 1):A275.

[18] Fleisch H. Bisphosphonates: mechanisms of action. Endocr Rev 1998;19(1):80–100.

[19] Zaidi M, Blair HC, Moonga BS, et al. Osteoclastogenesis, bone resorption, and osteoclast-based therapeutics. J Bone Miner Res 2003;18(4):599–609.

[20] Green JR. Bisphosphonates: preclinical review. Oncologist 2004;9(Suppl 4):3–13.

[21] Selby PL, Young MJ, Boulton AJ. Bisphosphonates: a new treatment for diabetic Charcot neuroarthropathy? Diabet Med 1994;11(1):28–31.

[22] Anderson JJ, Woelffer KE, Holtzman JJ, et al. Bisphosphonates for the treatment of Charcot neuroarthropathy. J Foot Ankle Surg 2004;43(5):285–9.

[23] Pitocco D, Ruotolo V, Caputo S, et al. Six-month treatment with alendronate in acute Charcot neuroarthropathy: a randomized controlled trial. Diabetes Care 2005;28(5):1214–5.

[24] Zaidi M, Inzerillo AM, Moonga BS, et al. Forty years of calcitonin—where are we now? A tribute to the work of Iain Macintyre, FRS. Bone 2002;30(5):655–63.

[25] Bem R, Jirkovska A, Fejfarova V, et al. Intranasal calcitonin in the treatment of acute Charcot neuroosteoarthropathy: a randomized controlled trial. Diabetes Care 2006;29(6):1392–4.

[26] Simonet WS, Lacey DL, Dunstan CR, et al. Osteoprotegerin: a novel secreted protein involved in the regulation of bone density. Cell 1997;89(2):309–19.

[27] Khosla S. Minireview: the OPG/RANKL/RANK system. Endocrinology 2001;142(12):5050–5.

Clin Podiatr Med Surg
25 (2008) 71–79

CLINICS IN
PODIATRIC
MEDICINE AND
SURGERY

Physical Management
of the Charcot Foot

Ryan T. Crews, MS*, James S. Wrobel, DPM, MS

*Center for Lower Extremity Ambulatory Research (CLEAR), Dr. William M. Scholl College
of Podiatric Medicine at Rosalind Franklin University of Medicine and Science,
3333 Green Bay Road, North Chicago, IL 60064, USA*

According to recent World Health Organization figures, 171 million people worldwide are afflicted with diabetes and this number is expected to climb to an astounding 366 million by 2030 [1]. Among the numerous sequelae associated with this disease, one of the worst and most common is diabetic foot ulceration. It has been estimated that the lifetime incidence rate of diabetic foot ulcers may be as high as 25% within the population of people with diabetes [2]. Foot ulcers provide an avenue for infection within the lower extremity, which may lead to the necessity of amputation of the lower extremity [3,4]. The proportion of individuals with ulcers who require at least a partial amputation is approximately 11% to 24% [5].

Although there are a number of risk factors associated with diabetes that predispose individuals to ulceration, peripheral neuropathy is typically the critical factor. Diabetic foot ulcers develop in response to the stresses placed on the plantar surface of the foot. Individuals with intact protective sensation in the feet may consciously or unconsciously alter their activity in response to stresses imparted to their feet. Without the sensation of pain, neuropathic individuals do not detect the inflammation and eventual autolysis of soft tissue beneath bony prominences of the foot [6,7]. Therefore, their first sign of trouble is often visual observance of a fully developed ulcer. To make matters worse, in some individuals neuropathy leads to Charcot arthropathy. This condition may cause anatomical remodeling of the foot that results in increased pressure at the midfoot [8], thereby increasing the likelihood of ulceration at that site [9,10].

The two prevailing and nonexclusive theories on the pathogenesis of Charcot arthropathy are the neurotraumatic and neurovascular theories

---

* Corresponding author.
E-mail address: ryan.crews@rosalindfranklin.edu (R.T. Crews).

doi:10.1016/j.cpm.2007.10.009   *podiatric.theclinics.com*

[11–13]. The neurovascular theory is based on a neurological and vascular interaction that results in excessive resorption of bone. The neurotraumatic theory asserts that an initial traumatic lesion of bone, cartilage, capsule, ligament, and/or tendon insertion in a neuropathic foot is necessary to initiate Charcot arthropathy [12,14,15]. "Continued weightbearing without the use of defensive strategies such as guarding, offloading, or limitation of activity propels the course and magnifies the intensity of the Charcot event" (p. 953) [12]. The continued application of stress on the foot and ankle leads to fracture and/or dislocation of the foot and ankle skeletal structure. As stress to the foot is a key initiator of Charcot arthropathy, the physical management of this condition is of utmost importance. In a retrospective study on patients with midfoot Charcot arthropathy, Pinzur [16] reported that more than half of these patients may be successfully treated by physical management without the need for surgery. The purpose of this manuscript is to review and discuss the physical management of the Charcot foot.

Progression of Charcot arthropathy

The goal of the physical management of Charcot arthropathy is to minimize stress to the foot by reducing shear forces and peak pressure, and redistributing the loads applied to the foot [17]. This, in turn, will limit the damage to the skeletal structure and soft tissue of the foot. The appropriate means to limit foot stress varies with the stage of Charcot arthropathy progression. The Eichenholz [18] classification system is a commonly used three-stage classification system based on clinical, radiographic, and pathologic data.

Stage I represents the development stage. Charcot arthropathy is initiated with an initial trauma followed by continued weight bearing over a period of weeks or months [16]. The initial injury may not be visible with plain radiographs but may be seen with an MRI as bone marrow edema [14]. Erythema, warmth, and swelling of the joints develop within the foot following the injury. The final step in the stage is fragmentation of bones within the foot. The most common site of fragmentation is at the tarsometatarsal (LisFranc) joint (40% to 48%), followed by Chopart's joint (30% to 34%) [19,20].

Stage II is referred to as the coalescent stage. During this stage the swelling, warmth, and erythema decrease and the destruction of bone comes to a halt [11,12]. The coalescent stage is marked by radiographic signs of early healing, with new bone formation and coalescence or fusion of larger fragments with adjacent bone [11].

Stage III is termed the reconstruction-consolidation stage. At this time the deformity fuses into a fixed and stable state [12]. Comparing the temperature gradient between the site of Charcot arthropathy and the same anatomic location on a healthy contralateral foot is a simple way to confirm radiographic signs of resolution. Armstrong and Lavery [21] found that elevated temperature at the site of Charcot arthropathy decreases in a predictable manner with the Charcot foot coming to mirror the healthy foot's temperature as acute arthropathy resolves. If the arch has collapsed during the acute phase, the bone permanently "heals" in this position. "The Charcot foot is the most extensive manifestation of neuro-osteoarth-opathy of the foot," (p. 484) [14] in which osteoarticular destruction of weightbearing bones and joints results in an inverted arch and rocker bot-tom sole. The modified anatomy of the foot results in increased pressure within the midfoot [8]. Fig. 1 displays the pressure profile of healthy foot

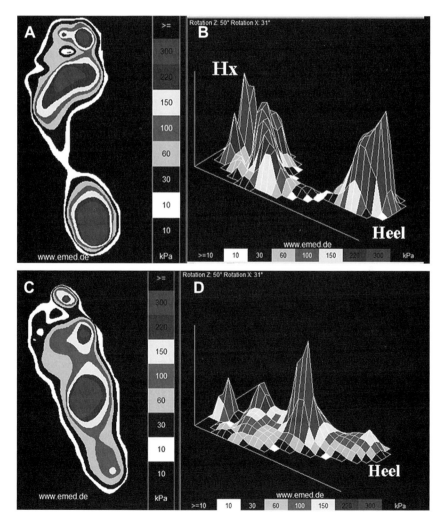

Fig. 1. Two-dimensional (2-D) and 3-D depiction of peak pressure of a single step with a healthy foot (*A* and *B*) and 2-D and 3-D depiction of peak pressure of a single step with a Charcot arthropathy–induced collapsed arch (*C* and *D*). Hx, Hallux.

(A and B) with peaks at the heel, metatarsal heads, and hallux. It also demonstrates the profile of a Charcot foot (C and D) with a large pressure spike within the midfoot. The result of the altered anatomy and pressure distribution of the foot is a subsequent increased risk of ulceration [9,22].

Physical management in stage I

The relationship between peak plantar pressure and the initiation of Charcot arthropathy was substantiated by Armstrong and Lavery [22] when they demonstrated that individuals in stage I have elevated peak pressures. Further evidence of the role of mechanical stress in the development of Charcot arthropathy was provided by Kimmerle and Chantelau [23]. They investigated the association between unrestrained weight bearing after a nonfracture injury and the development of Charcot deformities in patients with diabetic neuropathy. Individuals who were off-loaded (reduction in stress) early by means of total contact cast (TCC) were able to heal without deformities. However, the longer an individual partook in unrestrained weightbearing activity, the higher the risk of skeletal deformities (depressed or collapsed arch).

The TCC (Fig. 2) is considered the gold standard in initial treatment of Charcot arthropathy [12,20,23]. A TCC uses a well-molded, minimally padded cast, which maintains contact with the entire plantar surface of the foot and the lower leg [24]. By maintaining contact with the entire plantar surface, the cast disperses pressure across the entire foot, thereby minimizing isolated areas of high pressure or off-loading the foot. In the past off-loading and immobilization of a swollen pain-insensitive foot was not conducted

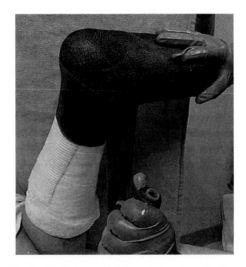

Fig. 2. Final stage of total contact cast application.

before the radiographic observance of fractures [14]. However, recent studies have indicated that by immediately off-loading feet that have suffered nonfracture bone injuries visible by MRI (bone bruise and bone marrow edema), one may prevent or minimize fractures and permanent deformities [14,23,25].

The TCC does have some drawbacks for care providers. Many centers do not have the infrastructure, expertise, or personnel to apply TCCs [26]. An alternative to the TCC is the instant total contact cast (iTCC) [27]. The iTCC (Fig. 3) simply consists of a commercial removable cast walker (Fig. 4) rendered irremovable by a layer of cohesive bandage, Elastoplast, or casting tape [24]. Removable cast walkers have been shown to be equivocal to total contact casts for the reduction of plantar pressure [28,29]. However, for the treatment of diabetic ulcers, removable cast walkers do not prove as effective as traditional TCC [30]. The difference in healing has been associated with poor compliance of walker use [31]. When walkers have been converted to iTCC the healing rate is improved [32]. In fact, an equivocal healing rate to that seen with TCC is achieved [33]. If a removable cast walker is used during stage I of Charcot arthropathy, we highly recommend that it be rendered irremovable to limit structural damage.

Physical management in stage II

As the clinical signs of swelling, warmth, and erythema decrease and the destruction of bone comes to a halt, patients may progress from a TCC or

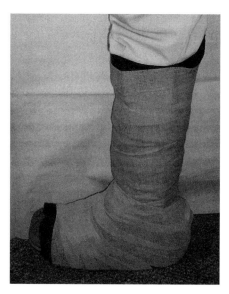

Fig. 3. Instant total contact cast.

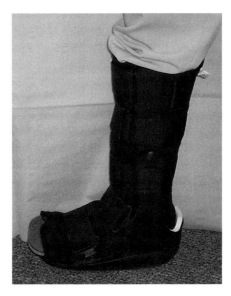

Fig. 4. Removable cast walker.

iTCC to a removable cast walker [20,21]. While using a walker, patients should be instructed to only remove it while sleeping or bathing. The mean time required for combined TCC and removable cast walker use has been reported to be 3 to 6 months [19,34]. However, Pinzur and colleagues [34] have suggested that prolonged TCC care is often necessary because of insufficient immobilization caused by infrequent cast changes that do not keep pace with decreases in swelling.

Physical management in stage III

With stage III, the focus of care transitions from minimizing skeletal structure remodeling to prevention of deformity-instigated ulceration [12]. Diabetic foot ulcers develop in response to excessive pressure and shear forces applied to the foot. Ulceration is common beneath the cuboid and cuneiform bones following Charcot arthropathy–induced skeletal remodeling. Commercially available extra-depth shoes (Fig. 5) in collaboration with custom-molded orthoses should sufficiently protect individuals with little or no deformation [12,15,19]. Severe foot deformities or remodeled ankles may require an ankle foot orthosis (AFO) or Charcot Restraint Orthotic Walker (CROW) [12,19]. An unstable or maligned rearfoot will benefit from a patellar tendon-bearing brace (PTB) and custom shoe [19].

Although the surgical management of Charcot arthropathy is not the focus of this piece, it should be noted that even with surgical reconstruction of Charcot alterations, accommodative footwear will be necessary as

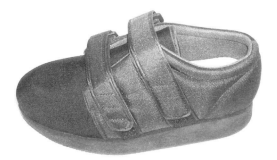

Fig. 5. Extra-depth shoe.

weightbearing loading of the foot will still be abnormal. Fig. 6 displays the pressure profile of the Charcot foot from Fig. 1 after receiving midfoot reconstruction involving an Achilles tenotomy and fusion of the tarsometatarsal joint. Although the large pressure spike at the midfoot is greatly relieved, there remains a small spike at the midfoot. Additionally, there is virtually no hallux contact with the ground, contributing to the large spike under the first metatarsal head. Furthermore, following panarthrodesis of Charcot ankles using intramedullary retrograde transcalcaneal nailing, Paola and colleagues [35] placed patients in shoes with a stiff rocker sole and molded insole to minimize foot stress.

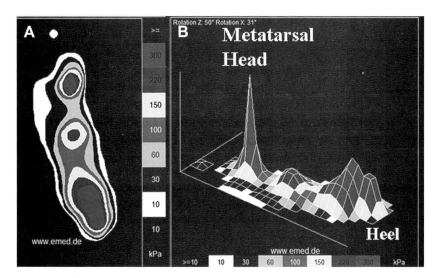

Fig. 6. Two-dimensional and 3-D depiction of peak pressure of a single step with of a surgically reconstructed Charcot foot (*A* and *B*).

Summary

The physical treatment of Charcot arthropathy is focused on the reduction of stress application to the skeletal structure of the foot and ankle. The appropriate treatment is dependent upon the progression of the condition. During stage I the standard treatment choice is the TCC. As the bone begins healing and the clinical signs of Charcot arthropathy diminish (stage II), care may be transitioned to a removable cast walker. When patients progress to the consolidation (stage III), providers should choose the most appropriate footwear as dictated by the severity of foot deformities. Among the many options available are extra-depth shoes, AFO, CROW, and PTB.

References

[1] World Health Organization. Diabetes programme. Available at: http://www.who.int/diabetes/en/. Accessed October 19, 2007.

[2] Singh N, Armstrong DG, Lipsky BA. Preventing foot ulcers in patients with diabetes. JAMA 2005;293(2):217–28.

[3] Armstrong DG, Lipsky BA. Advances in the treatment of diabetic foot infections. Diabetes Technol Ther 2004;6:167–77.

[4] Pecoraro RE, Reiber GE, Burgess EM. Pathways to diabetic limb amputation: basis for prevention. Diabetes Care 1990;13:513–21.

[5] LeMaster JW, Reiber GE. Epidemiology and economc impact of foot ulcers. In: Boulton AJM, Cavanagh PR, Rayman G, editors. The foot in diabetes. 4th edition. Chichester (England): John Wiley & Sons Ltd; 2006.

[6] Brand PW. The diabetic foot. In: Ellenberg M, Rifkin H, editors. Diabetes mellitus, theory and practice. 3rd edition. New York: Medical Examination Publishing; 1983. p. 803–28.

[7] Brand PW. The insensitive foot (including leprosy). In: Jahss M, editor. Disorders of the foot and ankle. 2nd edition. Philadelphia: Saunders; 1991. p. 2170–5.

[8] Wolfe L, Stess RM, Graf PM. Dynamic pressure analysis of the diabetic Charcot foot. J Am Podiatr Med Assoc 1991;81(6):281–7.

[9] Boyko EJ, Ahroni JH, Stensel V, et al. A prospective study of risk factors for diabetic foot ulcer. The Seattle Diabetic Foot Study. Diabetes Care 1999;22(7):1036–42.

[10] Armstrong DG, Wu SC, Crews RT. Algorithms for assessing risks for ulcerations and amputations. In: Boulton AJM, Cavanagh PR, Rayman G, editors. The foot in diabetes. 4th edition. Chichester: John Wiley & Sons Ltd.; 2006.

[11] Trepman E, Nihal A, Pinzur MS. Current topics review: Charcot neuroarthropathy of the foot and ankle. Foot Ankle Int 2005;26(1):46–63.

[12] Pinzur MS. Current concepts review: Charcot arthropathy of the foot and ankle. Foot Ankle Int 2007;28(8):952–9.

[13] Chantelau E, Onvlee GJ. Charcot foot in diabetes: farewell to the neurotrophic theory. Horm Metab Res 2006;38(6):361–7.

[14] Chantelau E, Richter A, Ghassem-Zadeh N, et al. "Silent" bone stress injuries in the feet of diabetic patients with polyneuropathy: a report on 12 cases. Arch Orthop Trauma Surg 2007; 127(3):171–7.

[15] Chantelau E, Kimmerle R, Poll LW. Nonoperative treatment of neuro-osteoarthropathy of the foot: do we need new criteria? Clin Podiatr Med Surg 2007;24(3):483–503.

[16] Pinzur M. Surgical versus accommodative treatment for Charcot arthropathy of the midfoot. Foot Ankle Int 2004;25(8):545–9.

[17] Saltzman CL, Hagy ML, Zimmerman B, et al. How effective is intensive nonoperative initial treatment of patients with diabetes and Charcot arthropathy of the feet? Clin Orthop Relat Res 2005;(435):185–90.

[18] Eichenholz SN. Charcot joints. Springfield (IL): Charles C. Thomas; 1966.

[19] Frykberg RG, Zgonis T, Armstrong DG, et al. Diabetic foot disorders. A clinical practice guideline (2006 revision). J Foot Ankle Surg 2006;45(5 Suppl):S1–66.

[20] Armstrong DG, Todd WF, Lavery LA, et al. The natural history of acute Charcot's arthropathy in a diabetic foot specialty clinic. Diabet Med 1997;14:357–63.

[21] Armstrong DG, Lavery LA. Monitoring healing of acute Charcot's arthropathy with infrared dermal thermometry. J Rehabil Res Dev 1997;34:317–21.

[22] Armstrong DG, Lavery LA. Elevated peak plantar pressures in patients who have Charcot arthropathy. J Bone Joint Surg Am 1998;80(3):365–9.

[23] Kimmerle R, Chantelau E. Weight-bearing intensity produces charcot deformity in injured neuropathic feet in diabetes. Exp Clin Endocrinol Diabetes 2007;115(6):360–4.

[24] Wu SC, Crews RT, Armstrong DG. The pivotal role of offloading in the management of neuropathic foot ulceration. Curr Diab Rep 2005;5(6):423–9.

[25] Chantelau E. The perils of procrastination: effects of early vs. delayed detection and treatment of incipient Charcot fracture. Diabet Med 2005;22(12):1707–12.

[26] Armstrong DG, Wu SC, Crews RT. New casting techniques: introduction to the 'instant total contact cast'. In: Boulton AJM, Cavanagh PR, Rayman G, editors. The foot in diabetes. 4th edition. Chichester (England): John Wiley & Sons Ltd; 2006.

[27] Armstrong DG, Short B, Nixon BP, et al. Technique for fabrication of an "instant" total contact cast for treatment of neuropathic diabetic foot ulcers. J Am Podiatr Med Assoc 2002;92:405–8.

[28] Lavery LA, Vela SA, Lavery DC, et al. Reducing dynamic foot pressures in high-risk diabetic subjects with foot ulcerations. A comparison of treatments. Diabetes Care 1996; 19(8):818–21.

[29] Baumhauer JF, Wervey R, McWilliams J, et al. A comparison study of plantar foot pressure in a standardized shoe, total contact cast, and prefabricated pneumatic walking brace. Foot Ankle Int 1997;18:26–33.

[30] Armstrong DG, Nguyen HC, Lavery LA, et al. Off-loading the diabetic foot wound: a randomized clinical trial. Diabetes Care 2001;24(6):1019–22.

[31] Armstrong DG, Lavery LA, Kimbriel HR, et al. Activity patterns of patients with diabetic foot ulceration: patients with active ulceration may not adhere to a standard pressure offloading regimen. Diabetes Care 2003;26(9):2595–7.

[32] Armstrong DG, Lavery LA, Wu S, et al. Evaluation of removable and irremovable cast walkers in the healing of diabetic foot wounds: a randomized controlled trial. Diabetes Care 2005;28(3):551–4.

[33] Katz IA, Harlan A, Miranda-Palma B, et al. A randomized trial of two irremovable off-loading devices in the management of plantar neuropathic diabetic foot ulcers. Diabetes Care 2005;28(3):555–9.

[34] Pinzur MS, Lio T, Posner M. Treatment of Eichenholtz stage I Charcot foot arthropathy with a weightbearing total contact cast. Foot Ankle Int 2006;27(5):324–9.

[35] Paola LD, Volpe A, Varotto D, et al. Use of a retrograde nail for ankle arthrodesis in Charcot neuroarthropathy: a limb salvage procedure. Foot Ankle Int 2007;28(9):967–70.

ELSEVIER
SAUNDERS

Clin Podiatr Med Surg
25 (2008) 81–94

CLINICS IN
PODIATRIC
MEDICINE AND
SURGERY

Surgical Management of Charcot Midfoot Deformities

Nicholas J. Bevilacqua, DPM*, Lee C. Rogers, DPM

Foot and Ankle Surgery, Amputation Prevention Center, Broadlawns Medical Center, 1801 Hickman Road, Des Moines, IA 50314 USA

Jean-Martin Charcot first described bone and joint changes in patients with syphilis and neuropathy in 1868. It was not until 1936 that W.R. Jordan established an association with Charcot arthropathy and diabetes mellitus. Today, it is well recognized that this syndrome can occur in conjunction with any peripheral neuropathy.

Charcot neuroarthropathy is a rapidly progressive and debilitating complication among persons with diabetes and may lead to gross deformity, ulceration, and amputation.

Charcot neuroarthropathy and the subsequent foot and ankle deformities negatively impact the lifestyle of the affected individual and may lead to permanent disability and premature retirement [1]. Early diagnosis and intervention is paramount and is associated with a significant lower incidence of deformity, in contrast to a delay in diagnosis and intervention [2]. Charcot neuroarthropathy is frequently misdiagnosed, often resulting in a delay in treatment resulting in worsening outcomes. Pakarinen and colleagues [3] reviewed 36 cases of Charcot neuroarthropathy and found the diagnostic delay averaged 29 weeks. These patients may or may not recall a traumatic event and present with erythema, warmth, and edema to the lower extremity resembling cellulites or acute septic arthritis. Frequently, they are given antibiotics and continue to ambulate on the affected foot and cumulate mechanical trauma in the acute phase results in significant bone and joint destruction.

Classification and joint involvement

In 1966, Eichenholtz [4] classified the sequence of changes in "Charcot joints" observed by means of serial radiographs and divided these changes

---

* Corresponding author.
  E-mail address: nicholas.bevilacqua@gmail.com (N.J. Bevilacqua).

0891-8422/08/$ - see front matter © 2008 Elsevier Inc. All rights reserved.
doi:10.1016/j.cpm.2007.10.007   *podiatric.theclinics.com*

into three stages: stage 1 (Stage of Development), stage 2 (Stage of Coalescence), and stage 3 (Stage of Reconstruction). Later, Shibata and colleagues [5] added an additional, earlier Stage 0, to Eichenholtz's classification, in which there are no radiographic changes noted, but there is warmth, swelling, and instability. Yu and Hudson [6] described Stage 0 as an acute sprain or fracture in the presence of neuropathy and reviewed the evaluation and treatment of this stage in the Charcot foot and ankle. Sella and Barrette [7] developed another classification scheme, also based on radiographic findings, which includes an early phase consisting of localized heat and swelling.

Sanders and Frykberg [8] developed an anatomic classification including involvement in the forefoot (pattern 1), the tarsometatarsal joint (pattern 2), the naviculocunieform and midtarsal joints (pattern 3), the ankle joint (pattern 4), and the posterior calcaneous (pattern 5). They found the midfoot (patterns 2 and 3) to be the most common area of involvement and often associated with plantar ulceration. Similarly, Brodsky and Rouse [9] described three types of joint involvement, the midfoot (type 1), the hindfoot (type 2), and the ankle (type 3) and noted the midfoot is involved 60% to 70% of the time. Schon and colleagues [10] developed a classification system categorizing acquired midtarsus deformities and concluded that midtarsus deformities can be classified as one of four types and one of three stages.

Treatment

In patients presenting with an acute Charcot neuroarthropathy with no apparent foot deformity, aggressive conservative treatment is the mainstay of therapy. Offloading, protection, and stabilization are the key components of therapy [11]. Often patients require a prolonged period of immobilization with a total contact cast (TCC) [12] or an instant total contact cast (iTCC). Armstrong and colleagues [13] treated 55 patients with Charcot neuroarthropathy with serial contact casting until quiescent and noted the duration of casting to be 18.5 weeks (± 10.6 weeks). Immobilization is continued until edema and temperature have subsided and radiographic signs of union are present [14]. Dermal thermometry [11] and serial radiographs are useful in monitoring the disease progression. A prompt and uncompromising offloading plan is often coupled with medical management. The recent recognition of the involvement that receptor activator of nuclear factor kappa B ligand (RANK-L) has in the osteolysis found in Charcot has led to the development of targeted therapy [15]. Researchers have demonstrated the benefits of intranasal calcitonin and found that its use reduced bone turnover by acting directly on the RANK-L signaling pathway in patients with acute Charcot neuroarthropathy [16].

At times, a patient may present with an unstable foot deformity that is difficult to accommodate. These patients frequently have a history of plantar foot ulcerations (Fig. 1). Failure to address the forces resulting in the deformity places the patient at risk for ulcer recurrence. In a study of 115 patients

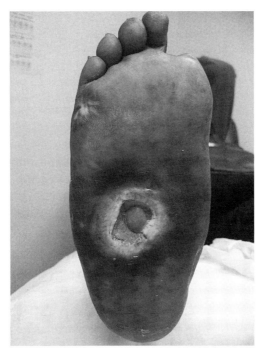

Fig. 1. Patient presenting with Charcot neuroarthropathy of the midfoot with an associated, nonhealing plantar foot ulceration.

(127 limbs) with a 3.8-year median follow-up, Saltzman and colleagues [17] noted a 2.7% amputation rate and a 49.0% ulcer recurrence rate after intensive conservative treatment of Charcot foot and ankle deformity. These patients frequently present with multiple fractures and dislocations with collapse of the midfoot being most common [8,9], resulting in a rockerbottom foot with increased plantar forefoot peak pressures and shearing forces. In this situation, accommodation and medical management alone are inadequate and surgical intervention is required. Midfoot deformities can be complex and may be associated with an open wound. In a structurally malaligned foot with an ulceration, the most important goal is to restore a stable, plantigrade foot with ulcer healing and elimination of infection [18]. Mitigating focal areas of increased pressure and shearing forces reduces the risk of ulcer recurrence. Foot and ankle reconstruction with external fixation has been shown to be an effective method of correcting the deformity and providing a stable, plantigrade, foot [19–22].

Principles of surgical reconstruction

As with any surgical candidate, a thorough history and physical are warranted. Persons presenting with Charcot neuroarthropathy often have multiple comorbidities and are morbidly obese. Patients must be medically fit and deemed appropriate candidates for the surgery and postoperative demands. Age, medical comorbidities, renal and cardiovascular status, nutritional status, and social history must be considered. Tight preoperative glycemic control is important in potentially reducing the risks for postoperative complications [23]. Preoperative education is imperative and if external fixation is planned, the surgeon should demonstrate how the device will appear on the patient's leg and the patient should be aware of the potential complications and prolonged recovery time. The goals of surgery should be clear to the patient and the surgeon before surgery and it is important to define an acceptable outcome. A favorable outcome has been defined as the ability to remain ulcer free and maintain walking independence in commercially available depth-inlay shoes with custom orthoses [19].

Physical examination often reveals the anatomic region of deformity. The surrounding skin and soft tissue is inspected and if an ulceration is present, osteomyelitis must be ruled out and eradicating soft tissue infection takes priority and should be controlled before surgery. Clinical inspection and radiographic analysis are used to determine the extent and stage of deformity. In patients presenting in the acute stage with deformity, the authors defer surgery until the edema and warmth subside. These patients are kept non-weightbearing in a Jones compressive-type bandage and are monitored with dermal thermometry. Only when the affected limb is within 4°F of the contralateral limb is surgery performed.

The degree of instability and adjacent joint range of motion are evaluated. Ankle range of motion must be assessed, as ankle equines is a pathologic component of midfoot collapse [24]. Weightbearing radiographic evaluation should include measurements of the lateral talar–first metatarsal angle, the calcaneal–fifth metatarsal angle, and the anteroposterior (AP) talar–first metatarsal angle (Fig. 2). Templates are helpful in planning osteotomies and bone resection needed to correct the deformity at the time of the surgery (Fig. 3) [25]. The correction is maintained with an external ring fixator. The ring sizes are determined and the device is prebuilt to include two tibial rings and one foot plate (Fig. 4).

External fixation is a logical choice when treating the Charcot midfoot deformity, as it does not rely on adequate bone stock [20]. Bone mineral density is reduced in patients with Charcot neuroarthropathy [26]. In this situation, it is unrealistic to expect internal fixation alone to maintain compression across the arthrodesis site and fixation failure with loss of correction is common (Fig. 5). The use of newer generation locking plates may be used in conjunction with external fixation [27]. External fixation provides uniform compression and allows for placement of fine wires away from the diseased bone. As mentioned earlier, Charcot midfoot deformities often present with an associated ulceration and unlike internal fixation, which use is cautioned when ulcerations are present, external fixation allows for continued access to the soft tissue throughout the recovery period (Fig. 6).

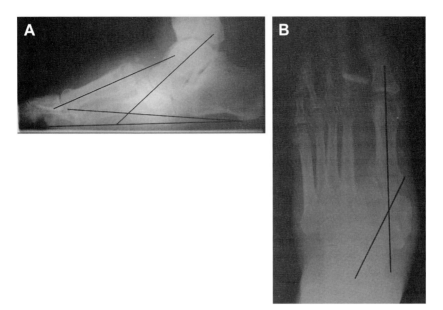

Fig. 2. (*A*) Weightbearing lateral radiographic demonstrating talar-first metatarsal angle and calcaneal-fifth metatarsal angle. (*B*) Weightbearing AP radiograph demonstrating talar-first metatarsal angle.

Surgical technique

Patients are placed in a supine position on the operating room table with the leg in a neutral position. General or regional anesthesia is obtained. A pneumatic thigh tourniquet is applied and the lower extremity is prepped and draped in the usual manner. An equinus deformity at the ankle is a key contributor to the collapse at this anatomical level and the hindfoot equinus is addressed with a percutaneous triple hemisection to reestablish the calcaneal inclination angle (Fig. 7). In cases of severe equines, the authors have

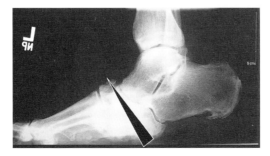

Fig. 3. Template used to determine the amount of bone resection required to correct deformity. Most midfoot deformities require a biplanar wedge with the apices lateral and dorsal.

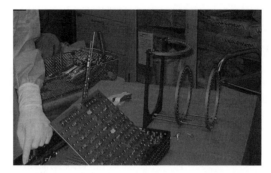

Fig. 4. Example of a prebuilt circular frame used for Charcot midfoot reconstruction includes two tibia rings and a foot plate.

performed an Achilles tenotomy to improve the calcaneal inclination angle and relieve the stress on the midfoot. If contracture still remains, a posterior ankle joint capsule release is performed.

Next, an incision is made medially at the apex of the deformity in line with the medial column. Subperiosteal dissection is carried laterally, carefully avoiding injury to the dorsalis pedis. A separate lateral incision may be placed if the planned bone resection involves the entire width of the forefoot. Malleable retractors are placed dorsal and plantar in preparation for bone resection (Fig. 8). A biplanar wedge of bone at the apex of the deformity is planned with the apices lateral and dorsal. For accurate resection of the biplanar wedge, Kirschner wires may be placed to guide the saw cut from medial to lateral. A sagittal saw is used to begin the bone cuts and the osteotomy is completed with an osteotome and mallet. The wedge of bone is removed (Fig. 9) and any defects may be filled in with autogenous bone or a bone graft substitute. The forefoot is stabilized to the hindfoot with two 4-mm Steinman pins. Reduction is directly visualized using intraoperative fluoroscopy (Fig. 10). Exact anatomic reduction is not required. A linear talar-first metatarsal relationship in transverse and sagittal planes

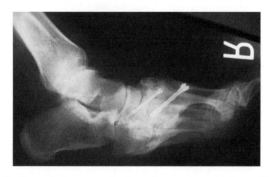

Fig. 5. Radiograph demonstrating loss of correction with internal fixation.

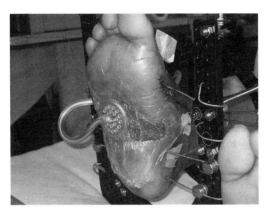

Fig. 6. Obtaining skeletal stabilization with the use of external fixation, while having direct access to the plantar foot ulceration. This case demonstrates the adjunctive use of negative pressure wound therapy.

with elimination of bony prominences generally result in a clinically planti-grade foot. When reduction is deemed satisfactory, the wounds are closed in layers over a drain. The tourniquet is deflated and the fixator is applied next.

At this point, the prebuilt frame consisting of two tibia rings and a foot plate are positioned on the foot and lower leg. The rings are centered on the limb ensuring adequate clearance between the skin and frame. Generally, two fingerbreadths anterior and three finger breaths posterior are sufficient to allow for postoperative edema. With placement of all wires, it is important to respect the anatomical safe zones and avoid penetration into neurovascu-lar structures. Wires are manually advanced through the soft tissue and power instrumentation is used to advance the wire through bone. As the wire passes the far cortex, a mallet is used to advance the wire through the remaining soft tissue and skin to reduce thermal necrosis around the wire.

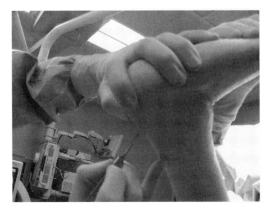

Fig. 7. Percutaneous triple hemisection performed to lengthen the Achilles tendon.

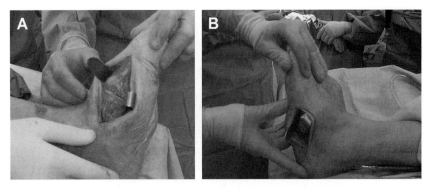

Fig. 8. (*A*) Intraoperative photograph demonstrating medial incision located at the apex of the midfoot deformity. (*B*) Intraoperative photograph of lateral incision. Note the malleable retractors placed dorsal and plantar in preparation for bone resection.

The calcaneus is initially stabilized with two tensioned olive wires placed at approximately 30 degrees to each other. Next, the frontal plane proximal and distal tibia wires are placed from lateral to medial perpendicular to the long axis of the tibia (Fig. 11). It is important to ensure bicortical purchase to prevent fracture through the bone. The wires are secured to the frame and tensioned accordingly. Next, wires are placed medial to lateral across the medial face of the proximal and distal tibia at approximately 45 degrees to their respective frontal plane wire (Fig. 12). These wires are secured to the ring and tensioned. At this point, one or two wires are placed proximal to the arthrodesis site and fastened to the foot plate and tensioned. Next, with the assistance of intraoperative fluoroscopy, a wire is placed in the forefoot distal to the osteotomy and "walked back" and secured to the foot plate one or two holes proximal to where it exited the foot (Fig. 13). As the wire is tensioned to the frame, the forefoot segment compresses against

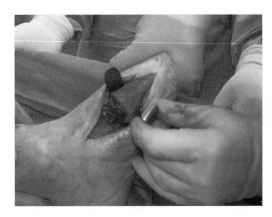

Fig. 9. Intraoperative photograph after resecting a biplanar wedge from the midfoot.

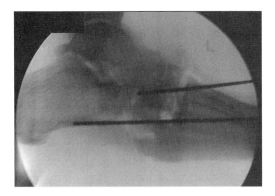

Fig. 10. Intraoperative fluoroscopy after stabilizing the forefoot to the hindfoot demonstrating a linear talar-first metatarsal with elimination of plantar prominence.

the hindfoot. This "bent-wire" technique allows for uniform compression at the arthrodesis site (Fig. 14).

Postoperative care

After a brief hospitalization, patients are sent home or preferably to a rehabilitation facility. The first dressing change is typically performed 5 to 7 days postoperatively and weekly thereafter. Pin care consists of povidine-iodine soaked 2 × 2-inch gauze with a pin slit cut into it. The authors have also found ease in using silver silicone foam (Mepilex Ag, Molylncke)

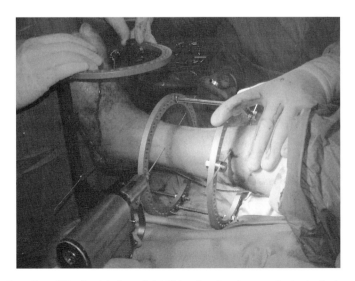

Fig. 11. Insertion of the frontal plane distal tibia wire placed perpendicular to the long axis of the bone.

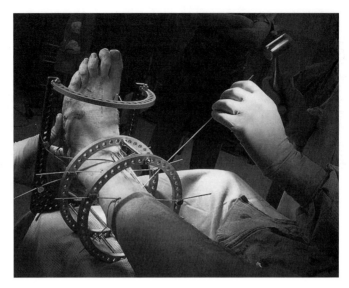

Fig. 12. Insertion of the proximal tibia wire placed across the medial face of the tibia at approximately 45 degrees to the frontal plane proximal tibia wire.

in dressing the pin sites. Again, the foam is cut in to 2 × 2-inch pieces and pin slits are cut into them. The silicone "sticks" to the skin and absorbs drainage, the silver ions neutralize bacteria, and the foam provides some compression. Patients are kept non-weightbearing and use either a wheelchair or a Roll-A-Bout (Roll-A-Bout Corporation, Frederica, DE) for ambulation. Patients receive deep vein thrombosis prophylaxis.

The external fixator is removed when clinical and radiographic evidence of consolidation is noted at the fusion site (Fig. 15). Typically, the frame is

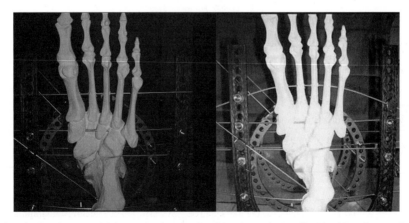

Fig. 13. Saw bone model demonstrating the distal forefoot wire "walked back" and secured to the foot plate one or two holes proximal to where it exited the foot.

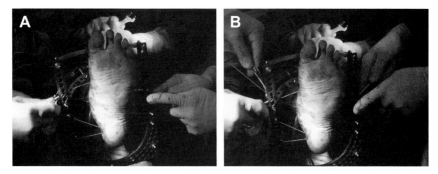

Fig. 14. (*A*) Intraoperative photograph demonstrating the "bent wire" technique. This picture was taken just before tensioning the wire. Note the arch in the wire. (*B*) Intraoperative photograph after tensioning the wire. The arched wire straightens as it is tensioned. This technique allows for uniform compression across the entire arthrodesis site.

removed after 10 to 12 weeks and patients are fitted for a Charcot Restraint Orthotic Walker (CROW) and remain in this device for up to 6 months (Fig. 16). After, patients are fitted for a commercially available extra-depth inlay shoe and are seen every 2 to 3 months for follow-up evaluation (Fig. 17).

Complications

Complications with Charcot reconstruction using external fixation are common and could be divided into minor and major complications. Minor

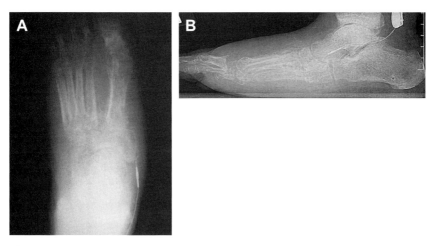

Fig. 15. (*A*) Postoperative AP radiograph after frame removal demonstrating osseous fusion at the midfoot and a linear talar-first metatarsal angle. (*B*) Postoperative lateral radiograph after frame removal demonstrating osseous fusion at the midfoot. Note the linear talar-first metatarsal angle and elimination of plantar prominence.

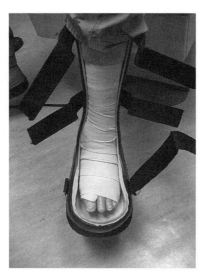

Fig. 16. Example of a CROW used for approximately 6 months after frame removal.

complications do not alter the postoperative course and include superficial wound dehiscence, wire irritation, or loss of wire stability. Major complications alter the postoperative course and, at times, require return trips to the operating room. These include soft tissue infections, wire breakage, and, most commonly, pin tract infections. The reported incidence of pin tract infection ranges between 5% and 100%, with most studies reporting in the range of 10% to 20% [23]. Erythema and drainage around pin sites are usually the result of micromotion or unstable wires and this may require wires to be tensioned further during the postoperative course to prevent further irritation and the development of a pin tract infection. Risk of postoperative

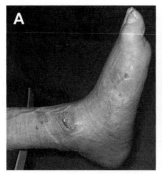
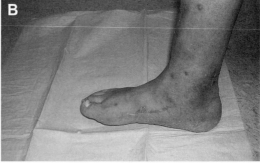

Fig. 17. (A, B) Clinical presentation of two patients 6 months after undergoing Charcot midfoot reconstruction with a favorable outcome. Both patients remain ulcer free in commercially available shoes.

infection is higher when reconstruction is performed in the presence of an open ulceration [28].

Risk of delayed union or nonunion is elevated in this high-risk population. The risk may be decreased with the use of an implantable bone stimulation device in these patients [29]. Smoking has been associated with an increased rate of nonunion and patients are offered assistance in quitting preoperatively.

Discussion

Diagnosing Charcot neuroarthropathy requires a heightened index of suspicion. Early recognition and intervention can limit deformity. Aggressive conservative management should be initiated early in the treatment plan in an effort to minimize the devastating effects often seen with this condition. Any patient with neuropathy presenting with even a minor foot and ankle injury should be immobilized and monitored closely. Dermal thermometry and serial radiographs are useful in monitoring the course of therapy. Conservative therapy is effective if initiated early in the treatment plan; however, any delay in therapy can result in severe foot and ankle deformity in which traditional nonoperative methods alone may be inadequate. These deformities may lead to ulcerations and ultimately progress to amputation of the lower extremity. Surgical correction and stabilization is an effective method to prevent further deformity and ulcer recurrence. Numerous studies have reported success with arthrodesis of the Charcot midfoot deformity with fusion rates ranging from 78% to 100% [30]. Pinzer [19] reported a 92% favorable outcome in 26 patients who underwent reconstruction for a high- risk, non-plantigrade Charcot midfoot deformity with a neutral ring fixator. Farber and colleagues [22] reviewed 11 patients with midfoot Charcot neuroarthropathy and ulceration. The patients underwent reconstruction with external fixation and all patients progressed to therapeutic footwear at an average 24-month follow-up. If performed in the appropriate setting and for the right indications, Charcot foot reconstruction is a better alternative to lower limb amputation.

References

[1] Pinzur MS, Evans A. Health-related quality of life in patients with Charcot foot. Am J Orthop 2003;32(10):492–6.

[2] Chantelau E. The perils of procrastination: effects of early vs. delayed detection and treatment of incipient Charcot fracture. Diabet Med 2005;22(12):1707–12.

[3] Pakarinen TK, Laine HJ, Honkonen SE, et al. Charcot arthropathy of the diabetic foot. Current concepts and review of 36 cases. Scand J Surg 2002;91(2):195–201.

[4] Eichenholtz SN, editor. Charcot joints. Springfield (IL): Charles C. Thomas; 1966;3–8.

[5] Shibata T, Tada K, Hashizume C. The results of arthrodesis of the ankle for leprotic neuroarthropathy. J Bone Joint Surg 1990;72A:749–56.

[6] Yu GV, Hudson JR. Evaluation and treatment of stage 0 Charcot's neuroarthropathy of the foot and ankle. J Am Podiatr Med Assoc 2002;92(4):210–20.

[7] Sella EJ, Barrette C. Staging of Charcot neuroarthropathy along the medial column of the foot in the diabetic patient. J Foot Ankle Surg 1999;38(1):34–40.

[8] Sanders LJ, Frykberg RG. The charcot foot. In: Frykberg, editor. The highrisk foot in diabetes mellitus. New York: Churchill Livingstone; 1991. p. 325–35.

[9] Brodsky JW, Rouse AM. Exostectomy for symptomatic bony prominences in diabetic Charcot feet. Clin Orthop Relat Res 1993;296:21–6.

[10] Schon LC, Easley ME, Weinfeld SB. Charcot neuroarthropathy of thefoot and ankle. Clin Orthop Relat Res 1998;349:116–31.

[11] Armstrong DG, Lavery LA. Acute Charcot's arthropathy of the foot and ankle. Phys Ther 1998;78:74–80.

[12] Pinzur MS, Lio T, Posner M. Treatment of Eichenholtz stage I Charcot foot arthropathy with a weightbearing total contact cast. Foot Ankle Int 2006;27(5):324–9.

[13] Armstrong DG, Todd WF, Lavery LA, et al. The natural history of acute Charcot's arthropathy in a diabetic foot specialty clinic. Diabet Med 1997;14:357–63.

[14] Baravarian B, Van Gils CC. Arthrodesis of the Charcot foot and ankle. Clin Podiatr Med Surg 2004;21(2):271–89.

[15] Jeffcoate W. Vascular calcification and osteolysis in diabetic neuropathy—is RANK-L the missing link? Diabetologia 2004;47(9):1488–92.

[16] Bem R, Jirkovska A, Fejfarova V, et al. Intranasal calcitonin in the treatment of acute Charcot neuroosteoarthropathy: a randomized controlled trial. Diabetes Care 2006;29(6):1392–4.

[17] Saltzman CL, Hagy ML, Zimmerman B, et al. How effective is intensive nonoperative initial treatment of patients with diabetes and Charcot arthropathy of the feet? Clin Orthop Relat Res 2005;(435):185–90.

[18] Garapati R, Weinfeld SB. Complex reconstruction of the diabetic foot and ankle. Am J Surg 2004;187(5A):81S–6S.

[19] Pinzur MS. Neutral ring fixation for high-risk nonplantigrade Charcot midfoot deformity. Foot Ankle Int 2007;28(9):961–6.

[20] Cooper PS. Application of external fixators for management of Charcot deformities of the foot and ankle. Semin Vasc Surg 2003;16(1):67–78.

[21] Wang JC, Le AW, Tsukuda RK. A new technique for Charcot's foot reconstruction. J Am Podiatr Med Assoc 2002;92(8):429–36.

[22] Farber DC, Juliano PJ, Cavanagh PR, et al. Single stage correction with external fixation of the ulcerated foot in individuals with Charcot neuroarthropathy. Foot Ankle Int 2002;23(2):130–4.

[23] Rogers LC, Bevilacqua NJ, Frykberg RG, et al. Predictors of postoperative complications of Ilizarov external ring fixators in the foot and ankle. J Foot Ankle Surg 2007;46(5):372–5.

[24] Armstrong DG, Peters EJ. Charcot's arthropathy of the foot. J Am Podiatr Med Assoc 2002; 92(7):390–4.

[25] Schon LC, Easley ME, Cohen I, et al. The acquired midtarsus deformity classification system–interobserver reliability and intraobserver reproducibility. Foot Ankle Int 2002;23(1):30–6.

[26] Petrova NL, Foster AV, Edmonds ME. Calcaneal bone mineral density in patients with Charcot neuropathic osteoarthropathy: differences between Type 1 and Type 2 diabetes-Diabet Med 2005;22(6):756–61.

[27] Weinraub GM. Midfoot arthrodesis using a locking anterior cervical plate as adjunctive fixation: early experience with a new implant. J Foot Ankle Surg 2006;45(4):240–3.

[28] Clohisy DR, Thompson RC. Fractures associated with neuropathic arthropathy in adults who have juvenile-onset diabetes. J Bone Joint Surg 1988;70A:1192–200.

[29] Saxena A, DiDomenico LA, Widtfeldt A, et al. Implantable electrical bone stimulation for arthrodeses of the foot and ankle in high-risk patients: a multicenter study. J Foot Ankle Surg 2005;44(6):450–4.

[30] Hockenbury RT, Gruttadauria M, McKinney I. Use of implantable bone growth stimulation in Charcot ankle arthrodesis. Foot Ankle Int 2007;28(9):971–6.

ELSEVIER
SAUNDERS

Clin Podiatr Med Surg
25 (2008) 95–120

CLINICS IN
PODIATRIC
MEDICINE AND
SURGERY

Surgical Reconstruction of the Charcot Rearfoot and Ankle

Patrick R. Burns, DPM, FACFAS[a,b,c],*,
Dane K. Wukich, MD[a,b,c]

[a]*Foot and Ankle Division, University of Pittsburgh School of Medicine, Roesch-Taylor Medical Building, North Suite 7100, 2100 Jane Street, Pittsburgh, PA 15203, USA*
[b]*Podiatric Surgical Training Program, University of Pittsburgh Medical Center South Side Hospital, 2000 Mary Street, Pittsburgh, PA 15203, USA*
[c]*University of Pittsburgh Medical Center, Comprehensive Foot and Ankle Center, Roesch-Taylor Medical Building, North Suite 7100, 2100 Jane Street, Pittsburgh, PA 15203, USA*

Destructive changes in the joints of patients who have neuropathy were described by Jean-Martin Charcot [1] in 1868 and later were described in the diabetic foot and ankle in 1936 by Jordan [2]. Peripheral neuropathy is universally present in patients who develop Charcot fracture/dislocation, and the number of patients who have diabetes and associated peripheral neuropathy is on the rise [3,4].

Other factors play a role, however. An area currently under investigation at the cellular level is receptor activator of nuclear factor kappa B ligand. Normal regulation and counterbalance of osteoclasts and osteoblasts may be altered in the patient who has peripheral neuropathy and may cause the loss in structural integrity and subsequent failure [5]. The history and pathophysiology are reviewed more thoroughly in other articles in this issue.

Although the exact mechanism is not known, the ultimate goal of treatment, whether nonoperative or operative, is to achieve a stable, plantigrade foot. Achieving this status is challenging in the rearfoot and ankle. Statistically, Charcot deformity affects the rearfoot and ankle less often than the midfoot, but the resultant deformities typically are more severe and difficult to stabilize conservatively. The resultant instability in the ankle leads to a limb-threatening deformity, and surgical intervention and salvage are

---

* Corresponding author. Foot and Ankle Division, University of Pittsburgh School of Medicine, Roesch-Taylor Medical Building, North Suite 7100, 2100 Jane Street, Pittsburgh, PA 15203.
E-mail address: burnsp@upmc.edu (P.R. Burns).

doi:10.1016/j.cpm.2007.10.008

more common. To date, few data on the best course of treatment are available, but the use of limb-salvage techniques is on the rise. With increasing knowledge of the disease and with technological advances in internal and external fixation, limb salvage is becoming more consistent. This article discusses basic techniques in deformity planning and current uses of internal and external fixation techniques for rearfoot and ankle limb salvage.

Diagnosis, staging, and classification

In many cases the traumatic event that initiates Charcot changes goes unrecognized. This lack of recognition can delay the diagnosis and can affect treatment. At least 25% of cases have improper or delayed diagnosis, and some studies show even higher rates [6,7].

Radiographic findings of Charcot deformity are well known. Destruction of bone and joint, debris, dislocation, and osteopenia are common findings; however, they may not be present initially. Clinical suspicion should remain high when warmth, edema, and erythema present in the neuropathic patient (Fig. 1). Most often this presentation is unilateral and commonly is misdiagnosed as gout, infection, or deep venous thrombosis. Bilateral events are less likely but are reported in approximately 10.4% of patients [8]. In any event, foot and ankle surgeons must continually educate patients and other health care providers about these subtle findings and Charcot deformity.

Infection must be ruled out in patients who have an open ulcer or a history of previous surgery. Without a portal of entry, it is unlikely that the increased erythema and temperature localized to the foot or ankle would result from infection. A thorough examination of the skin for loss of skin integrity and evaluating the patient for fevers, chills, and a change in glycemic control is paramount. Patients who have acute Charcot deformity manifest local signs of inflammation without the typical systemic signs of increased white cell count or fever. A simple test of elevating the leg for

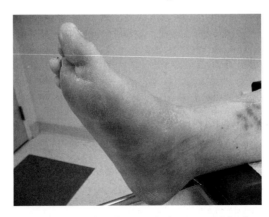

Fig. 1. Typical clinical presentation of erythema and edema seen with a foot with acute Charcot deformity.

10 minutes should show decrease in the edema in a patient who has Charcot deformity, whereas the edema will persist in infection [9].

If the patient has a wound, the proper steps need to be taken. Local care, off-loading techniques, imaging studies, deep cultures, and biopsies aid in the diagnosis. Nonhealing ulcers or those that show no improvement with standard care should be examined more thoroughly, and surgical intervention often is necessary (Fig. 2). Intraoperative debridement allows proper cultures and specimens to be sent for analysis to determine the presence and number of white cells. Bone can be sampled as well for diagnosis of osteomyelitis. Charcot deformity and infection can coexist, and proper diagnosis is needed to guide treatment. Intraoperative frozen sections and infectious disease consultations help guide antibiotic therapy.

Vascular status must also be evaluated properly. Noninvasive studies are now recommended yearly in patients who have diabetes, independent of subjective complaints. In the patient who has neuroarthropathy, the ankle brachial index typically demonstrates adequate flow. Studies show the ankle brachial index in patients who have Charcot deformity average 0.65 during the process [10–13]. This finding still needs to be regarded with caution, because diabetic patients have both macro- and microvascular disease, making the interpretation of these tests challenging.

The classic radiograph of Charcot deformity is identified easily because few disease processes have such a profound effect with widespread dislocation and debris (Fig. 3). Osteomyelitis is a common misdiagnosis because of the bone destruction and periosteal reaction. Differentiation of Charcot deformity from osteomyelitis may be difficult radiographically, especially when a wound is present. There continues to be debate about the best modality for differentiating osteomyelitis from Charcot arthropathy. MRI is very sensitive in showing marrow edema and abscess, but others believe indium-labeled white cell scans are more reliable for distinguishing between the two conditions [10,11,14].

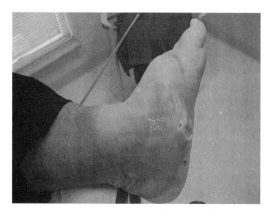

Fig. 2. Talar dislocation and ulceration associated with acute Charcot deformity of the ankle.

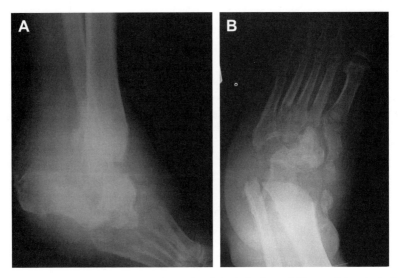

Fig. 3. (*A*) Lateral and (*B*) oblique radiographs of classic findings of Charcot deformity including dislocation, destruction, and debris.

Radiographs are critical for staging, classification, and defining treatment options. Traditionally, surgery during the acute stage has not been recommended because of poor results. Staging systems became useful in treatment protocols, and Eichenholtz [15] in 1966 was the first to classify three stages. Charcot deformity progresses through what he determined were well-defined developmental, coalescence, and remodeling stages. These stages were easily identifiable and aided in treatment planning. He believed that surgery would have better results if performed either in early stage 1 or late stage 3, presumably because of relatively less inflammation and overall increased stability and structural integrity of bone.

Harris and Brand [16] followed this idea and suggested that arthrodesis be performed early in the disease process. Similarly, Newman [17] found that early arthrodesis and a period of immobilization of the involved joint could prevent further deformity. This practice was not widely adopted, however; others noted hardware failure and infection, so early surgical intervention has not been recommended for treating the initial stages. Traditionally stage 1 has been treated with conservative measures including total contact casting and off-loading. Surgery was reserved for the more predictable later stage 3. There are no comparative or prospective studies for definitive guidance.

The concept of Charcot stage 0 was later added by Shibata and colleagues [18] for the "at risk" patient who has neuropathy and injury. Presumably, these patients have a much higher chance of progressing to the destructive stages, even though initial radiographs are negative. If treated appropriately, the Charcot cycle would not progress to the destructive stage. This area has seen much interest recently, particularly in diabetic ankle fractures [19].

Because of increased complication rates, current recommendations are for more stable constructs, prolonged non–weight-bearing, and increased number of office visits to attempt to minimize the possibility of a Charcot event (Fig. 4).

Classification based on anatomy, inclusive of the entire foot and ankle, has been described by Brodsky [9,20] and by Sanders and Frykberg [21]. Schon and colleagues [22] also classified Charcot deformity with a focus on the midtarsus alone. The classifications based on location aid in treatment plans and prognosis. Deformities become less stable and more often require intervention with longer immobilization periods as they move proximal. The Brodsky and Sanders/Frykberg classifications differ in the actual "type" and location, but the overall statistics remain similar. Clearly the incidence of Charcot deformity in the midfoot makes up the majority in both systems (60% to 70% in Brodsky type 1, which includes the tarsometatarsal and naviculocuneiform joints). The Sanders/Frykberg classification including the same joints is considered type II and type III, comprising about 55% of cases. Although the classification systems do not match perfectly in location or joints involved, they do show overall similarities in the percentages of midfoot involvement. Corresponding types involving the ankle from both systems include Brodsky type 3a at 10% and Sanders/Frykberg type IV at 9%.

Hindfoot and ankle literature

Outcomes and evidenced-based medicine regarding Charcot ankle and hindfoot deformity is minimal. Most literature consists of case series or

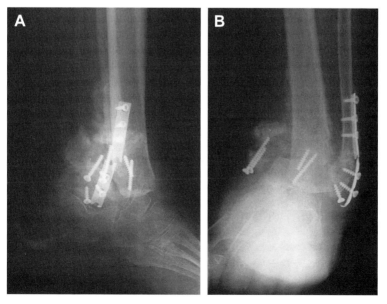

Fig. 4. (*A*) Lateral and (*B*) anteroposterior radiographs of a diabetic ankle fracture which converted to an acute Charcot deformity with subsequent hardware failure and deformity.

expert opinion. Midfoot Charcot deformity has been the focus of most studies of treatment and outcomes, presumably because of its greater incidence. Nonoperative treatments show acceptable outcomes in much midfoot Charcot literature, possibly because of the greater inherent stability of the region. Acute rearfoot and ankle Charcot deformity is less stable and is more likely to require surgery, but it also is overall less common than midfoot disease. There are no studies comparing conservative versus surgical treatment in the ankle or rearfoot, and the majority of the literature regarding rearfoot and ankle Charcot deformity is anecdotal or small, retrospective studies.

Today, increasing numbers of surgeons are beginning to advocate earlier intervention for Charcot changes [23,24]. In 2000, Simon and colleagues [25] published an arthrodesis study that demonstrated successful restoration of anatomic alignment with the use of open reduction internal fixation and fusion in the acute developmental stage of Charcot breakdown. Stable fusion was achieved in all 14 patients in this study of midfoot Charcot deformity. To date there are no similar studies concerning the acute event in the rearfoot or ankle, and more studies are needed before these types of surgery are considered routine or standard in the acute patient.

In midfoot disease, Pinzur [26,27] found approximately 60% of 147 patients at 1-year follow-up required no surgery and could be managed with shoe and brace modifications. The remaining 60 patients in the study required corrective surgery, mainly consisting of triple arthrodesis to address a nonplantigrade foot. In this retrospective review, eight amputations were performed on this group in the 1-year period. Pinzur [28] also reported on 237 patients in which the diagnosis of Charcot deformity was made over a 10-year period. Over that time period 120 patients required 143 operations. Surgeries ranged from debridement to major amputation. The article did not elaborate on location or classifications to stratify outcomes but did state that 55 ankle or hindfoot fusions were performed along with 21 major amputations. It did not give data to correlate location with these events or other complication rates specific to the ankle or hindfoot. This benchmark analysis was aimed more at projecting costs for the health care system to allocate resources appropriately.

Saltzman and colleagues [8] reviewed 127 limbs to determine survivorship and amputation rate. The actual number of major amputations was 15 of 127, giving an annual risk of 2.72 per 100 patients on a survivorship curve. This finding was similar to Pinzur's [28] benchmark review of 237 patients in which the overall amputation rate was 9%. In Saltzman's article [8] the location of Charcot deformity did not seem to affect the rate of amputation, but the numbers were too low to be significant. As expected, patients who had recurrent ulceration did show a significant increase in amputation rate, as did patients who presented initially with an ulceration compared with those who had an intact skin envelope. This study included Charcot deformity at every level, 32 of which were of the ankle or hindfoot requiring six major amputations. A majority of the surgery performed addressed midfoot pathology. A total of 53 non-amputation surgeries were performed, including two ankle fusions and three hindfoot fusions to address unstable deformities. There were no amputations in this surgically treated group.

Zarutsky and colleagues [29] reported on 43 patients undergoing salvage ankle arthrodesis with the use of external fixation. Eleven of those patients underwent surgery for Charcot reconstruction. The data and complications did not separate out the patients who had Charcot deformity from the others, but a major complication rate of 51.2% was noted for the series. Complications included abscess and non-union, and one of the two below-knee amputations reported in the series occurred in a patient who had Charcot deformity. Although this study was not exclusively of Charcot reconstruction, the complexity of external fixation for these salvage cases was expressed.

Papa and colleagues [13] reported on 29 patients; of these a large percentage had rearfoot and ankle involvement. The series reported on salvage with arthrodesis in 21 ankle and 6 subtalar joints with longstanding neuroarthropathy. It may be that this study contains a high number of rearfoot and ankle patients because these patients were less stable and so were less likely to respond to the typical conservative treatments, but this possibility was not discussed. The patients were operated on in later stages of the disease, and a variety of rearfoot and ankle fusions were performed as needed. Most received internal fixation with only four external fixators. The article does state ankle brachial index findings were a mean of 0.86, and some of the fusions were performed in the presence of a nonhealing wound. Sixty-six percent achieved a solid fusion at 5 months. The most likely fusion to develop a pseudoarthrosis was tibiocalcaneal, which fused in only 4 of 11 procedures. One patient was lost to follow-up, one patient underwent below-knee amputation, one patient had recurrent ulceration, and the remaining patients were successfully stabilized long term with bracing.

Internal fixation with intramedullary nail fixation in the treatment of Charcot ankle and rearfoot deformity was reviewed retrospectively by Caravaggi and colleagues [30]. Bracing had failed in 14 patients who had severe ankle instability. All ulcerations were healed before surgery was performed, and all surgeries took place in the later remodeling phase of Charcot deformity. In the end, the authors showed a 92.8% salvage rate, with unions in 10 of 14 patients. There were three fibrous unions that developed after hardware failure in the calcaneus and one below-knee amputation for osteomyelitis. This case series shows good results in patients who had late-stage Charcot deformity, affording the stability required in the ankle and rearfoot for ambulation with bracing.

There was a similar finding by Pelton and colleagues [31] using intramedullary retrograde nailing for salvage of ankle and rearfoot deformity. Ten of the 33 patients in the series had the diagnosis of Charcot deformity. The union rate for the entire series was 88%. There were four non-unions, two of which were in patients who had Charcot deformity, making non-union in the small Charcot subset 2 of 10. These non-unions remained stable and braceable, leading the authors to state they believe this technique is favorable in the Charcot reconstruction because of the increased stiffness compared with lag screws, especially when the distal screws are inserted posterior-to-anterior through the calcaneus.

Charcot deformity related to leprosy was reviewed by Shibata and colleagues [18]. In this series, 26 fusions were performed with intramedullary rod (17 ankle and 9 tibiocalcaneal) after talectomy. Most were performed in the later stages. Four, however, were performed in stage 0, and one was performed in stage 1. The authors achieved fusion in 73% (ie, 19 attempts); all their failures in the later stage 3 patients.

Fabrin and colleagues [32] reviewed 12 feet in 11 patients over a 12-year period in whom external fixation was used for management of Charcot ankle deformity. Most studies still lean toward internal fixation, but a recent trend toward external fixation can be seen. This study stated that external fixation was used because of the presence of ulceration and unstable deformity. There were seven tibiotalar fusions and five tibiocalcaneal fusions. Only one of these failed, leading to below-knee amputation, with 6 of the 12 going on to union. The remaining fibrous unions were stable and braceable. Four of the five fibrous unions were seen in the tibiocalcaneal patients. A Charnley-type device was used for fixation and was kept in place for 6 weeks, followed by an additional 6 weeks of total contact casting. The results in these salvages are similar to those reported for internal fixation techniques and are encouraging. This study in late-stage Charcot deformity with open wounds gives options to those trying to salvage these difficult patients. At the University of Pittsburgh, external fixators and non–weight-bearing periods are much longer, but a similar trend of a higher rate of fibrous union for tibiocalcaneal fusions is seen.

Stuart and Morrey [33] reported on ankle fusion in 13 diabetic patients, all of whom had a history of ankle trauma. Nine of the patients had evidence of neuroarthropathy radiographically. Only seven ankles achieved union. Three patients underwent amputations, two developed non-unions, and one patient died. External fixation was used in nine cases and internal fixation in four. Complication rates were high, with 20 re-operations, leading the author to conclude that caution should be used in the neuropathic ankle. There was no correlation between location or method of fixation and failure, but neuropathy did correlate with poor results.

Ligament laxity and soft tissue instability were discussed by Brink and colleagues [34], along with a case study concerning a talar dislocation with Charcot deformity. This case was treated with a triple arthrodesis. The relevance was the mention and discussion of the soft tissue structures and their role. Clearly Charcot deformity is not only a bone disorder, and although it is easy to see the changes radiographically, failure occurs on many levels.

Moore and colleagues [35] reviewed 19 intramedullary rods for ankle arthrodesis. The study included rheumatoid and posttraumatic ankles, but the largest group had Charcot ankle deformities (seven patients). Overall there were five pseudarthroses, one infection, and one broken rod for the entire review population. Most patients required bracing afterwards, but none of the pseudarthroses had symptoms. The authors concluded that the use of an intramedullary rod should be considered for salvage, especially in cases of bone loss and osteopenia such as neuropathic arthropathy.

Myerson and colleagues [36] reviewed internal fixation of the neuropathic ankle using an adolescent condylar blade plate with allograft bone in 30 patients, 26 of whom had diabetic neuroarthropathy with talar fragmentation. Many of these patients were offered amputation as an alternative, many had undergone multiple prior surgeries, and eight had previous osteomyelitis. Many of these patients had ulcerations at the time of surgery. The surgery was performed with removal of remaining talus and placement of morcelized bone graft with antibiotic powder to fill the void. A rigid plate then was applied. Fusion was achieved in 28 of 30 patients on average of 16 weeks. Besides the two non-unions, there were two stress fractures at the proximal plate and three superficial infections. This review was a continuation of a report of Alvarez and colleagues' [37] use of a condylar plate for fusion of a neuropathic ankle in seven patients. The mixture of allograft and antibiotics was used in all seven of these patients and resulted in 100% union at 5.2 months.

Principles of therapy

Although there is much debate about treatment types and timing, the end goal is the same. Stable chronic patients are monitored and off-loaded as needed (Fig. 5). If a patient presents in the acute stages of neuroarthropathy, conversion to the later more "quiet" stages is a primary concern. During that time, maintaining structure or limiting further collapse is of extreme importance. This goal can be accomplished initially by total contact casting, the use of Charcot restraint orthotic walkers, or plain non–weight-bearing. Each of these modalities has its own difficulties, from nonadherence to instructions to iatrogenic ulceration. It can be quite difficult for some patients to use crutches and perform a three-point gait, and doing so can predispose the contralateral limb to high pressures and even Charcot events [38].

If reasonable alignment is maintained, therapy is continued without change. On the other hand, if significant collapse continues during the initial visits, a decision needs to be made about correction and the timing of correction, which can reduce the chance of ulceration or aid in its healing. Relieving the deformity and therefore its pressure is a common reason for performing Charcot reconstruction. Reduction during the pliable acute stage and maintaining the reconstruction with external fixation until coalescence is becoming more common in attempted treatment.

Stability aids in wound healing and also may help in conversion to later stages of Charcot deformity. This conversion may be augmented with several

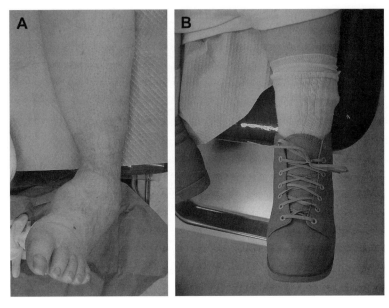

Fig. 5. Clinical pictures of a Charcot ankle deformity (*A*) before and (*B*) after surgical correction with accommodative shoes and bracing.

additional modalities. The natural history of Charcot deformity is to continue through its stages, with or without intervention. The questions are, what is the time frame involved, and how can it be expedited?

The use of electricity to aid in bone healing was described in the late 1800s, and bone's piezogenic properties were discovered in the late 1950s [39]. Later work in the 1960s showed electricity could induce new bone formation [40].

In the recent years, bone stimulation with pulsed electrical fields and low-intensity ultrasound has been described to aid in the repair of bone. This technique has been used mostly in cases of non-union or fusions. There have been few studies of bone stimulation in the foot and ankle and even fewer with regards to Charcot arthropathy [41–43]. A few studies do exist with Hanft [41] reporting on 31 patients who had acute stage 1 Charcot deformity. Two groups were formed, 10 control patients and 21 study patients. Time to consolidation was reduced in the study patients (11 weeks, versus 23.8 weeks for the control group), and there was less bony destruction in the study group. The groups were not broken down by the location of the Charcot event.

Acting on anecdotal reports or with expert opinion, many foot and ankle surgeons use a form of bone stimulation during the acute Charcot process with or without surgery, but evidence-based research is lacking.

Bisphosphonate therapy, which inhibits osteoclastic bone resorption, may be another adjunct to overall Charcot management. Studies of the use of a few of the bisphosphonates in patients who have Charcot deformity have shown some promising results [44–46]. During treatment, patients receiving these therapies showed decreases in markers of osteoclastic activity as well as local temperatures. How this experience correlates with clinical practice or with the location of deformity is not yet known.

Basic surgical principles

Preventing further deformity is a key element in the treatment of patients who have Charcot deformity. In many cases the acute Charcot event, if treated appropriately, can maintain reasonable alignment, and surgery or ulceration from pressure areas in the midfoot can be avoided [26]. This experience has not been described in rearfoot and ankle literature.

Acute or chronic deformity with instability often requires surgical stabilization. Acute Charcot deformity in the hindfoot and ankle leads to greater instability than in the midfoot; therefore the potential for major complication is higher. In the acute patient who has severe deformity and collapse, external fixation is used commonly, whether or not there is concomitant ulceration. Stability will aid the repair of soft tissues, much as in open trauma situations, and the external fixator allows access for local care. The fixator also may allow the correction and maintenance of deformity during the initial stages.

Often the acute deformity can be corrected on the table, held temporarily with large Steinman pins, and stabilized with an external fixator. Other cases require the use of olive wires and motors to help pull segments (Fig. 6). Still others with complex deformity and multiple centers of rotation of angulation (CORA) can be treated with advanced technology such as the Taylor's Spatial Frame (Smith and Nephew, Inc., Memphis, Tennessee), which allows continual computer-aided adjustment. To date no level 1 evidence supports these treatments or theories, although some articles describing techniques are available [47].

Internal fixation in the acute setting has been attempted, but hardware failure is common, especially if the fragmentation stage has occurred, presumably because of insufficient bone strength and the continuation of deformity. External fixation does allow further distribution of the body weight, fixation away from the acute diseased bone, and possibly more stable fixation in poor-quality bone. External fixation wires and pins also can be doubled to increase fixation and can be revised much more readily if needed.

With chronic deformity, ulceration is common. The first goal is to heal the ulceration with standard treatments including off-loading and local wound care. In the event of nonhealing or recurrent wounds, surgery can be performed [13]. Often the deformity itself is the main cause for the nonhealing ulceration and thus must be addressed. Preoperative planning, including templates and CORA measurements, becomes crucial. Osteotomies and bone wedge resection can correct deformity, with the surgeon's choice of fixation and local plastic techniques to aid in closure.

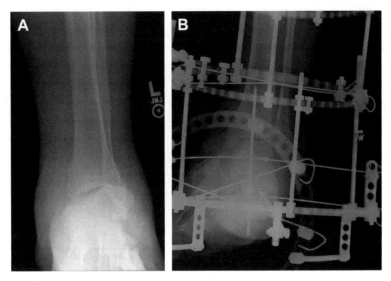

Fig. 6. (*A*) Acute Charcot deformity with subluxation of the ankle joint. (*B*) Closed reduction was performed with application of external fixation. An olive wire locked to a threaded rod was used to pull the talus medially reducing the ankle joint.

Surgical techniques

Equinus

The Charcot rearfoot and ankle deformity can be a difficult problem, frequently associated with multiple locations of deformity. One of the most common issues, and the easiest to identify, is the equinus contracture of the Achilles tendon. There is controversy about whether equinus has a causal relationship with Charcot joint deformities. Equinus increases stress on the medial arch and forefoot, but many patients who have equinus do not progress to Charcot arthropathy. In general, it is agreed that equinus contracture plays some role, and most Charcot reconstructions are performed with concomitant lengthening of the Achilles tendon or gastrocnemius.

Calcaneal inclination on lateral radiographs is a common way to identify equinus and can be used to assess equinus objectively. The normal calcaneal inclination is about 20° from the weight-bearing surface. In Charcot foot and ankle deformities, this angle is decreased significantly or even has a negative value (Fig. 7). As a sequela of the Achilles tendon contracture, the calcaneus loses its normal position, resulting in altered biomechanics and adjacent ligament and joint failure. In theory, lengthening of the Achilles tendon should help recover calcaneal inclination and take stress off the compensating joints. Lengthening of the Achilles tendon has been shown to decrease its power, decrease pressures on the midfoot and forefoot, and increase available dorsiflexion [48]. With these findings, there is no

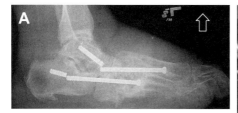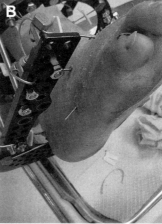

Fig. 7. (*A*) Complication of failed internal fixation. (*B*) Broken skinny wire of an external fixator.

measurable change in functional limitations in patients after Achilles lengthening [49]. Such findings lend support to the theory that midfoot collapse in many patients who have Charcot deformity is initiated by equinus.

Most of the changes that occur after lengthening are temporary, lasting 7 to 8 months, but at 2-year follow-up Mueller and colleagues [49] found the recurrence of midfoot ulcerations was 38%, compared with to 81% for total contact casting. Even though power and pressures returned many ulcerations remained healed.

A percutaneous technique with three-stab incisions is often preferred (Fig. 8). The initial incision is made parallel with the tendon, beginning just medial to its border and 2 cm proximal to the insertion. The blade is inserted and turned 90°, and the tendon is cut percutaneously by feel. Two similar stab incisions are made at 2-cm intervals more proximal along the tendon, alternating lateral and medial. The foot is dorsiflexed during the process until lengthening is achieved. (One must avoid overcorrection, which leads to a calcaneal gait. In the insensate patient, that gait can create the further complication of plantar heel ulcerations.) These incisions are small, and closure is not required.

Management of the chronic stage

Once conservative measures have failed to control the deformity, heal ulcerations, or provide a stable extremity amenable to bracing, surgical intervention is warranted. Osseous intervention in the rearfoot and ankle is challenging. Corrective osteotomies or tendon work alone will not give

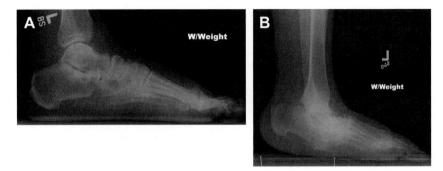

Fig. 8. Radiographs of (*A*) normal and (*B*) abnormal calcaneal inclination angle caused by Charcot deformity.

the needed long-term stability. As in other joints with Charcot deformities, arthrodesis is the treatment of choice, but achieving a solid fusion can be challenging. In a review of arthrodesis of the Charcot knee deformity, Drennan and colleagues [50] found that important factors for success include (1) careful removal of all cartilage and debris, (2) debridement to bleeding subchondral bone, (3) meticulous fashioning of bone surfaces for contact, (4) complete debridement of all synovial and scarred capsule, and (5) stable internal fixation.

There are many options for rearfoot and ankle fusions. Once the joints are prepared, unhealthy bone has been debrided, and the deformity has been corrected, the area is stabilized. Internal fixation uses large screws, plates, and intramedullary fixation. Increased stability can be achieved with locked plates, reconstruction plates, or blade plates.

Correction of osseous deformities requires preoperative and intraoperative planning and often requires templates (Fig. 9). In the operating room, the patient must be positioned properly. With rearfoot and ankle procedures, a bump under the ipsilateral hip with the patient in a supine position is most common. This position allows the leg to be in a more neutral position for deformity correction and also makes the lateral side more accessible for surgical approach to the ankle. The leg should be prepped and draped above the knee. Fixation for these deformities requires access to the entire leg. The knee is also a landmark for rotation of the lower extremity. To reduce the chance of malunion during arthrodesis, external rotation should align the second toe and the tibial crest. A thigh tourniquet commonly is used as well. In many cases, the tourniquet is elevated during the dissection and deformity correction to aid in visualization and is released once temporary fixation is in place.

Correction can be acute, staged, or partial with plans for continued gradual correction. There are no level 1 studies to guide these plans, but an understanding of biomechanics and knowledge of anatomy are crucial. Many of the resultant deformities are unique, but restoration of normal

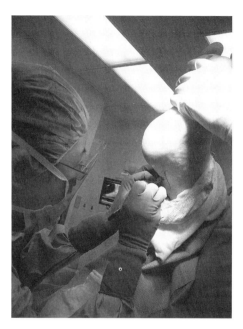

Fig. 9. Percutaneous Achilles lengthening.

anatomic relationships continues to be the cornerstone of management. It is helpful to draw out basic anatomy and common angles on the radiographs to determine the axis of rotation and apex of deformity. Knowledge of these relationships will guide the location and size of wedge resections. During the procedure, Kirschner wires are placed along the lines of the previously planned osteotomies and act as a guide. The saw and osteotomes then can follow along the wires, removing the appropriate bone.

Charcot ankle deformity, although representing only 5% of the deformities, results in unstable varus and valgus malalignment. Acute corrections of varus can compromise the tarsal tunnel. During acute varus corrections, prophylactic release of the tarsal tunnel should be considered. In general, any large correction of angle or length can cause vessels to kink, leading to ischemia. When there is large, acute loss of height, as in Charcot ankle deformity and talectomy, a more gradual, staged correction may be necessary.

Incisions are large. For the rearfoot and ankle, a utilitarian lateral incision often is used. It begins approximately 6 cm from the tip of the lateral malleolus, courses along the lateral border of the fibula, and then makes a gentle curve over the sinus tarsi and calcaneal cuboid joint. This incision allows access to much of the rearfoot and ankle complex. The fibula, if present, is removed 5 cm proximal to the ankle joint and can be used as graft if healthy. The ankle and subtalar joints are visualized easily, and talectomy can be performed if needed.

A second medial incision may be used. It typically is positioned just anterior to the medial malleolus and courses between the tibialis anterior and posterior tendons. This incision allows access to the talonavicular joint and medial gutter of the ankle for medialization of the talus for intramedullary rod fixation. Both incisions can communicate anteriorly, with dissection carried across the distal tibia. A malleable retractor can be used here to protect tissues during corrective osteotomies (Fig. 10).

After more "normal" relationships are established and deformity has been corrected, Steinman pins are used for temporary fixation across the rearfoot and ankle. Calcaneal inclination is one important key. Once the rearfoot and ankle are reduced, it gives a building block for the remaining midfoot, and ankle deformities can be addressed. Depending on final fixation, a half-pin is inserted into the calcaneus using fluoroscopy. It enters posteriorly following the normal inclination angle. After the Achilles lengthening, the half-pin can be used to pull the Achilles into a more anatomic position (Fig. 11). At this time a transfixation pin is placed and aids in holding the rearfoot. It enters the inferior calcaneus and is driven proximally through the talus, if present, and into the anterior cortex of the tibia (Fig. 12). These pins can be incorporated later into an external fixator, if used. Together these pins provide stability of the rearfoot during further correction. From this point the remaining fixation depends on surgeon preference, clinical circumstances, available healthy bone, and comfort level. Internal fixation is common. At the University of Pittsburgh Medical School external fixation is used frequently and may be used as an adjunct. External

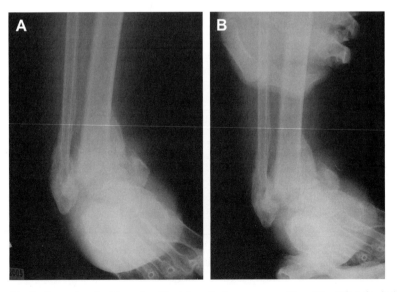

Fig. 10. Radiographs of a Charcot ankle deformity in a varus position. The deformity is (A) stressed and (B) clearly rigid, which is useful in preoperative planning.

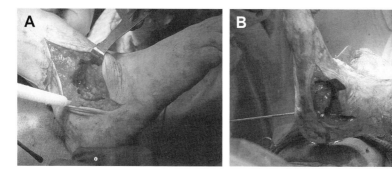

Fig. 11. Standard (*A*) lateral and (*B*) medial incisions for reconstruction of Charcot rearfoot and ankle deformity with a malleable retractor for protection of soft tissue.

fixation also can be used alone, especially in the face of open ulceration or the acute Charcot process, where fixation is needed away from the unhealthy neuropathic bone.

Whatever the type of fixation, the use of larger, sturdier, and even doubled hardware is common. For internal fixation, locking plates are available. With these plates, all components are locked together at a fixed angle, to disperse force better. For failure to occur, the entire construct must fail, not just one screw. Extra wires, half-pins, or full rings are some of the easiest ways to increase the strength of external fixation.

External fixation does have drawbacks. In a review of a consecutive series from the University of Pittsburgh Medical School, 60% to 70% of complications were minor and did not require a change in treatment, but they make this technique labor intensive and challenging.

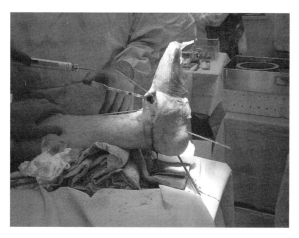

Fig. 12. Although for a midfoot reconstruction, this photograph shows the calcaneal half-pin used posteriorly to improve the inclination angle. A transfixation pin then was placed from inferior calcaneus into the tibia proximally.

Management of the acute stage

If the deformity is considered too unstable for conservative management in the acute phase, surgical options exist. Many principles remain the same. The patient in the operating room must be prepared similarly, and Achilles lengthening is performed in the standard fashion. Preoperative planning of deformity is essential. As in chronic deformities, the calcaneus is reduced under fluoroscopy and is pinned as described previously. The remaining correction of midfoot to rearfoot and rearfoot to ankle relationships can then be made.

In the acute phase, this correction may be achieved with manipulation and stabilized with Steinman pins. Fluoroscopy guides reduction, and fixation is applied. Other options include external fixation techniques with olive wires, washers, and motors. These devices can help reduce and then stabilize the dislocations (Fig. 13). Many of these corrections are made percutaneously to avoid making large incisions in unfavorable skin conditions.

Acute Charcot deformity can be reduced and maintained by external fixation, but long-term results are not available. As the patient continues through the Charcot stages, consolidation may occur and be held in place with the fixator, but the achievement of long-term stability usually requires definitive arthrodesis. Early surgical intervention, however, affords easier reduction in the supple phases so that staged arthrodesis is more anatomic and possibly easier to perform.

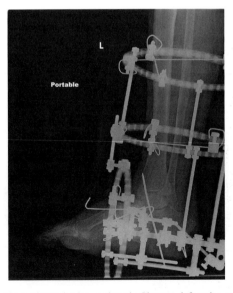

Fig. 13. Radiograph of a patient who has a chronic Charcot deformity undergoing reconstruction. The ankle and rearfoot were corrected and then held in place with a transfixation Steinman pin from the plantar aspect of the calcaneus into the anterior tibial cortex.

Whatever the fixation modality, long periods of non–weight-bearing and frequent office visits are necessary. A good support system for both the patient and surgeon are essential, because follow-up is labor intensive.

Case illustrations

Case 1

A 41-year-old woman who had type 2 diabetes and a history of increasing deformity over the past several months was referred for evaluation (Fig. 14). She had been treated by another physician with serial debridements and off-loading after obvious Charcot neuroarthropathy. Swelling, warmth, and erythema eventually calmed, and the wound finally closed, but during the postoperative follow-up the deformity could not be braced successfully. She eventually had a recurrence of ulceration that would not heal.

On clinical examination, she had a rigid rearfoot varus of 40° and a non-infected ulcer on the lateral weight-bearing foot. Radiographs showed remodeling stages of Charcot deformity with obvious varus deformity of the ankle and minimal talus remaining.

Surgically, the goal was to remove the varus and achieve a plantigrade foot and ankle to off-load the lateral column. A small acute correction of 15° was performed with an osteotomy through standard incisions. An external fixator was applied to correct the remaining deformity gradually to limit neurovascular compromise. The remaining varus was corrected over the next 3 weeks.

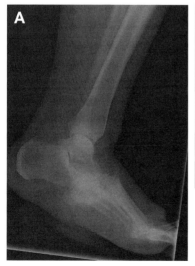
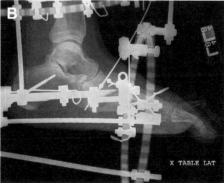

Fig. 14. Lateral radiograph of (*A*) an acute Charcot deformity with collapse and (*B*) percutaneous treatment with olive wires to improve medial column arch height.

Once a rectus ankle was achieved, long-term stability was achieved with a tibial-calcaneal fusion. An intramedullary rod was placed upon removal of the external fixator. The patient continues to wear custom shoes without recurrence. It has been the author's (PRB) experience that ankle and tibial-calcaneal fusions using an external fixation alone frequently are fibrous unions and revert back to some deformity once the fixator is removed. Therefore placement of an intramedullary rod after correction has become common.

Case 2

A 45-year-old man who had type 2 diabetes was well known to the author (PRB), who had treated the patient for previous Charcot events in the both feet (Fig. 15). A new, acute Charcot event with ulceration and drainage of the left ankle brought him through the emergency room.

Clinically he had a warm, erythematous ankle with obvious instability. The ulceration laterally with significant drainage was cultured. He was admitted, and radiographs and MRI revealed an acute Charcot process of the ankle, destruction of the talus, and abscess. This condition was treated with incision and drainage, biopsy, antibiotic beads, intravenous antibiotics, and external fixation for stability. After months of treatment with multiple debridements, biopsies, and antibiotics, a tibial-calcaneal fusion with bone graft was performed with intramedullary rod fixation. The graft was placed to limit acute loss of height after destruction of the talus. To date the patient remains stable in custom shoes and external upright braces.

Case 3

A 49-year-old man who had type 2 diabetes presented with a 6-week history of swelling and redness (Fig. 16). He had been treated for gout by his primary care physician after presenting following a "sprain." He was referred because of continued symptoms. Clinically no open wounds were noted, but significant erythema and edema around ankle was noted. The ankle had obvious instability and deformity on examination. Radiographs revealed a subluxed ankle and dislocated midfoot with Charcot changes. (Fig. 17)

He was admitted, and an external fixator was placed. The fixator allowed stability during the acute Charcot process but also permitted reduction of the dislocation and subluxation with minimal incisions. Once distracted, olive wires and motors were used to reduce the deformities.

During the next few months the ankle became infected, and the fixator was adjusted as needed with debridement of the ankle joint. Biopsies were taken, and appropriate antibiotics were given. The fixator was continually compressed over the ankle during this process along with the appropriate antibiotics. It was clear the talus would be lost, and the goal was a tibial-calcaneal fusion. As the patient progressed to later stages of Charcot

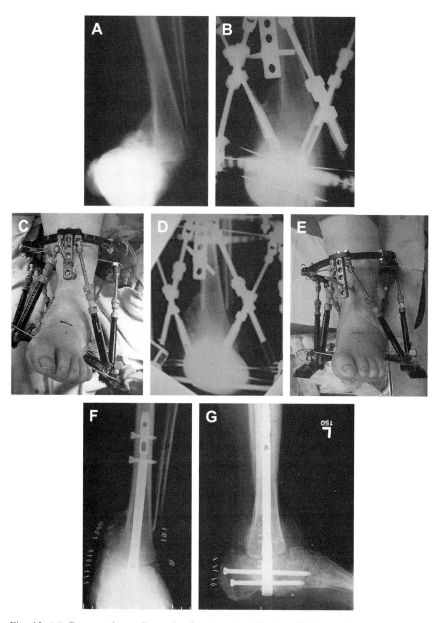

Fig. 15. (*A*) Preoperative radiograph of a chronic deformity. (*B*) Immediate postoperative radiograph and (*C*) clinical pictures. (*D*) Radiograph and (*E*) clinical pictures 3 weeks after gradual correction. (*F*, *G*) Final radiographs with intramedullary rod for fixation.

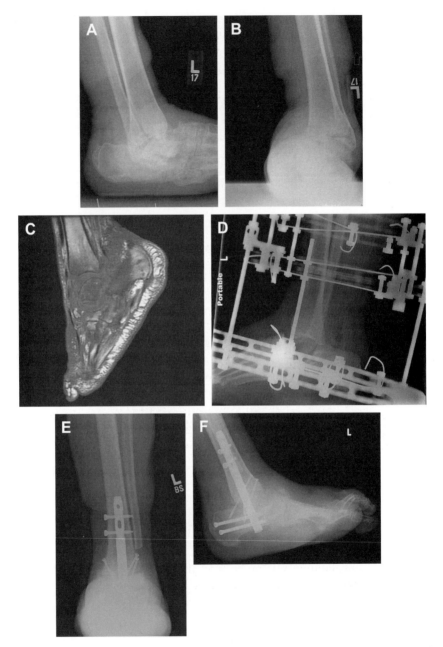

Fig. 16. (*A*, *B*) Preoperative radiographs of acute Charcot deformity. (*C*) MRI of abscess and Charcot deformity surrounding the talus. (*D*) External fixator during serial debridement and talectomy. (*E*, *F*) Postoperative radiographs after graft and intramedullary rod placement.

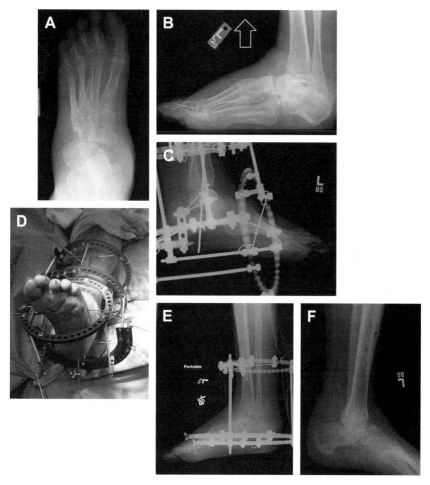

Fig. 17. (*A*, *B*) Preoperative radiographs of acute dislocation. (*C*) Radiograph and (*D*) clinical pictures of postoperative reduction with external fixator. Subsequent radiographs (*E*) after debridement with continued compression and stability with (*F*) stable outcome.

deformity, consolidation was noted, and the patient remained stable. The fixator was periodically compressed during the process and produced a stable fusion that is braced without further surgery required.

Summary

Charcot arthropathy of the rearfoot and ankle is a complex disorder. To date there are no evidence-based, universally agreed upon treatment protocols. Many propose earlier intervention of these acute deformities, but their treatment is challenging. As the number of patients who have these deformities continues to increase, surgeons' skill levels and experience grow as well. With increased technical skill, knowledge, and advances in fixation, these deformities are becoming more manageable. In the future this experience should afford the general community with evidenced-based protocols. These deformities are demanding and require a good support system for both the surgeon and patient, but a stable, braceable limb is obtainable.

Further readings

Sanders LJ, Frykberg RG. The high risk foot in diabetes mellitus. New York: Churchill-Livingstone; 1991.
Pinzur MS, Sage R, Stuck R, et al. A treatment algorithm for neuropathic (Charcot) midfoot deformity. Foot Ankle 1993;14(4):189–97.

References

[1] Charcot JM. [Sur quelques arthropathies. Qui paraissent dependre d'une lesion. Du cerveau ou de la moelle epiniere]. Arch Physiol Norm Pathol 1868;1:161–78 [in French].
[2] Jordan WR. Neuritic manifestations in diabetes mellitus. Arch Intern Med 1936;57:307–66.
[3] Armstrong DG, Lavery LA. Elevated peak plantar pressures in patients who have Charcot arthropathy. J Bone Joint Surg Am 1998;80(3):365–9.
[4] Lavery LA, Armstrong DG, Wunderlich RP, et al. Diabetic foot syndrome: evaluating the prevalence and incidence of foot pathology in Mexican American and non-Hispanic whites from a diabetes disease management cohort. Diabetes Care 2003;26(5):1435–8.
[5] Jeffcoate WJ, Game F, Cavanagh PR. The role of proinflammatory cytokines in the cause of neuropathic osteoarthropathy (acute Charcot foot) in diabetes. Lancet 2005;366(9502):2058–61.
[6] Schon LC, Marks RM. The management of neuroarthropathic fracture-dislocations in the diabetic patient. Orthop Clin North Am 1995;26:375–92.
[7] Chantelau E. The perils of procrastination: effect of early vs. delayed detection and treatment of incipient Charcot fracture. Diabet Med 2005;22:1707–12.
[8] Saltzman CL, Hagy ML, Zimmerman B, et al. How effective is intensive nonoperative initial treatment of patients with diabetes and Charcot arthropathy of the feet? 2005;(435):185–90.
[9] Brodsky JW. The diabetic foot. In: Mann RA, Coughlin MJ, editors. Surgery of the foot and ankle. St. Louis (MO): Mosby-Year Book; 1993. p. 877–958.
[10] Myerson MS, Edwards WH. Management of neuropathic fractures in the foot and ankle. J Am Acad Orthop Surg 1999;7:8–18.
[11] Myerson MS. Diabetic neuroarthropathy. In: Myerson MS, editor. Foot and ankle disorders. Philadelphia: W.B. Saunders; 2000. p. 439–65.
[12] Myerson MS, Papa J, Eaton K, et al. The total-contact cast for management of neuropathic plantar ulceration of the foot. J Bone Joint Surg Am 1992;74:261–9.
[13] Papa J, Myerson MS, Girard P. Salvage, with arthrodesis, in intractable diabetic neuropathic arthropathy of the foot and ankle. J Bone Joint Surg Am 1993;75-A(7):1056–66.
[14] Levine SE, Myerson MS. Management of ulceration and infection in the diabetic foot. In: Myerson MS, editor. Foot and ankle disorders. Philadelphia: W.B. Saunders; 2000. p. 411–38.
[15] Eichenholtz SN. Charcot joints. Springfield (IL): Charles C. Thomas; 1966.
[16] Harris JR, Brand PW. Patterns of disintegration of the tarsus in the anaesthetic foot. J Bone Joint Surg Br 1966;48(1):4–16.

[17] Newman JH. Non-infective diseases of the diabetic foot. J Bone Joint Surg Br 1981;63-B(4): 593–6.
[18] Shibata T, Tada K, Hashizume C. The result of arthrodesis of the ankle for leprotic neuro-arthropathy. J Bone Joint Surg Am 1990;72(5):749–56.
[19] Prisk VR, Wukich DK. Ankle fractures in diabetics. Foot Ankle Clin 2006;11(4): 849–63.
[20] Brodsky JW, Rouse AM. Exostectomy for symptomatic bony prominences in diabetic Charcot feet. Clin Orthop Relat Res 1993;296:21–6.
[21] Sanders LJ, Frykberg RG. Diabetic neuropathic osteoarthropathy. The Charcot foot. In: Frykberg RG, editor. The high risk foot in diabetes mellitus. New York: Churchill Living-ston; 1991. p. 297.
[22] Schon LC, Weinfeld SB, Horton GA, et al. Radiographic and clinical classification of acquired midtarsus deformities. Foot Ankle Int 1998;19(6):394–404.
[23] Wang JC. Use of external fixation in the reconstruction of the Charcot foot and ankle. Clin Podiatr Med Surg 2003;20(1):97–117.
[24] Pinzur MS, Stuck R, Sage R, et al. Benchmark analysis on diabetics at high risk for lower extremity amputation. Foot Ankle Int 1996;17(11):695–700.
[25] Simon SR, Tejwani SG, Wilson DL, et al. Arthrodesis as an early alternative to nonoperative management of Charcot arthropathy of the diabetic foot. J Bone Joint Surg Am 2000; 82A(7):939–50.
[26] Pinzur MS. Surgical versus accommodative treatment for Charcot arthropathy of the midfoot. Foot Ankle Int 2004;25(8):545–9.
[27] Pinzur MS, Lio T, Posner M. Treatment of Eichenhotlz stage 1 Charcot foot arthropathy with a weightbearing total contact cast. Foot Ankle Int 2006;27(5):324–9.
[28] Pinzur MS. Benchmark analysis of diabetic patients with neuropathic (Charcot) foot defor-mity. Foot Ankle Int 1999;20(9):564–7.
[29] Zarutsky E, Rush SM, Schuberth JM. The use of circular wire external fixation in the treat-ment of salvage ankle arthrodesis. J Foot Ankle Surg 2005;44(1):22–31.
[30] Caravaggi C, Cimmino M, Caruso S, et al. Intramedullary compressive nail fixation for the treatment of severe Charcot deformity of the ankle and rearfoot. J Foot Ankle Surg 2006; 45(1):20–4.
[31] Pelton K, Hofer JK, Thordarson DB. Tibiotalocaneal arthrodesis using a dynamically locked retrograde intramedullary nail. Foot Ankle Int 2006;27(10):759–63.
[32] Fabrin J, Larsen K, Holstein PE. Arthrodesis with external fixation in the unstable or mis-aligned Charcot ankle in patients with diabetes mellitus. Int J Low Extrem Wounds 2007; 6(2):102–7.
[33] Stuart MJ, Morrey BF. Arthrodesis of the diabetic neuropathic ankle joint. Clin Orthop Relat Res 1990;253:209–11.
[34] Brink DS, Eickmeier KM, Levitsky DR, et al. Subtalar and talonavicular joint dislocation as presentation of diabetic neuropathic arthropathy with salvage by triple arthrodesis. J Foot Ankle Surg 1994;33(6):583–9.
[35] Moore TJ, Prince R, Pochatko D, et al. Retrograde intramedullary nailing for ankle arthrod-esis. Foot Ankle Int 1995;16(7):433–6.
[36] Myerson MS, Alvarez RG, Lam PW. Tibiocalcaneal arthrodesis for the management of severe ankle and hindfoot deformities. Foot Ankle Int 2000;21(8):643–50.
[37] Alvarez RG, Barbour TM, Perkins TD. Tibiocalcaneal arthrodesis for nonbraceable neuro-pathic ankle deformity. Foot Ankle Int 1994;15(7):354–9.
[38] Lesko P, Maurer RC. Talonavicular dislocations and midfoot arthropathy in neuropathic diabetic feet. Natural course and principles of treatment. Clin Orthop Relat Res 1989;(240):226–31.
[39] Fukuda E, Yasuda I. On the piezoelectric effect of bone. J Physiol Soc Japan 1957;12: 1158–64.

[40] Bassett CA, Becker RO. Generation of electric potentials by bone in response to mechanical stress. Science 1962;137:1063–4.

[41] Hanft JR, Goggin JP, Landsman A, et al. The role of combined magnetic field bone growth stimulation as an adjunct in the treatment of neuropathy/Charcot joint: an expanded pilot study. J Foot Ankle Surg 1998;37(6):510–5.

[42] Bier RR, Estersohn HS. A new treatment for Charcot joint in the diabetic foot. J Am Podiatr Med Assoc 1987;77(2):63–9.

[43] Grady JF, O'Connor KJ, Axe TM, et al. Use of electrostimulation in the treatment of diabetic neuroarthropathy. J Am Podiatr Med Assoc 2000;90(6):287–94.

[44] Selby PL, Young MJ, Boulton AJ. Bisphosphonates: a new treatment for diabetic Charcot neuroarthropathy? Diabetic Med 1994;11(1):28–31.

[45] Jude EB, Selby PL, Burgess J, et al. Bisphosphonates in the treatment of Charcot neuroarthropathy: a double-blind randomized controlled trial. Diabetologia 2001;44(11):2032–7.

[46] Pitocco D, Ruotolo V, Caputo S, et al. Six-month treatment with alendronate in acute Charcot neuroarthropathy. Diabetes Care 2005;28(5):1214–5.

[47] Roukis TS, Zgonis T. The management of acute Charcot fracture-dislocations with the Taylor's spatial external fixation system. Clin Podiatr Med Surg 2006;23(2):467–83.

[48] Maluf KS, Mueller MJ, Strube MJ, et al. Tendon Achilles lengthening for the treatment of neuropathic ulcers causes a temporary reduction in forefoot pressure associated with changes in plantar flexor power rather than ankle motion during gait. J Biomech 2004; 37(6):897–906.

[49] Mueller MJ, Sinacore DR, Hastings MK, et al. Impact of Achilles tendon lengthening on functional limitations and perceived disability in people with a neuropathic plantar ulcer. Diabetes Care 2004;27(7):1559–64.

[50] Drennan DB, Fahey JJ, Maylahn DJ. Important factors in achieving arthrodesis of the Charcot knee. J Bone Joint Surg Am 1971;53-A(6):1180–93.

ELSEVIER
SAUNDERS

Clin Podiatr Med Surg
25 (2008) 121

CLINICS IN
PODIATRIC
MEDICINE AND
SURGERY

Current Therapy: Special Articles

ELSEVIER
SAUNDERS

Clin Podiatr Med Surg
25 (2008) 123–126

CLINICS IN
PODIATRIC
MEDICINE AND
SURGERY

The Cone Flap: A Fasciocutaneous Flap Option for Plantar Heel Ulcers

Andrew Rader, DPM, FACFAOM, CWS, FAPWCA[a,b,*],
Timothy Barry, DPM, AACFAS[a]

[a]Memorial Hospital and Healthcare Center, The Wound Care Center,
800 West 9th Street, Jasper, IN 47546, USA
[b]St. Mary's Healthcare Center, The Diabetic Foot Clinic, 3700 Washington Avenue,
Evansville, IN 47750, USA

Chronic plantar heel wounds present a difficult dilemma for the podiatric specialist. With the advent of vacuum-assisted closure devices and other advanced wound-healing modalities, getting a wound to epithelialization has become increasingly common. The wound healed by secondary intention on the plantar foot remains fragile, however. The authors have had success with more durable primary closure options for these wounds, including the reverse-flow sural fasciocutaneous flap, sural free flap, and local myofasciocutaneous flap using the abductor hallucis muscle belly with split-thickness plantar skin grafting. A limitation of these techniques is the specialized training required to perform them.

Fasciocutaneous flaps were first described by Poten [1] in 1981 as a way to raise a skin flap based on the vascular plexus of the underlying fascia. Since then, fasciocutaneous flaps have demonstrated reliable success in the clinical and experimental fields [2,3]. The fasciocutaneous system consists of perforating vessels arising from regional arteries that pass through the muscular layer along fibrous septa. The vessels then form plexi above and below the plane, which ultimately distribute perforating branches to the overlying skin [4]. Random skin flaps have a reliable length-to-width ratio of 1:1. Knowledge of the vascular supply from the fascia has enhanced that reliable ratio to between 2:1 and 3:1 [1]. The cone flap is a fasciocutaneous flap based on the vascular supply through the plantar fascia. Direct closure of the donor site is achieved using a combined technique of rotational flap and V-Y advancement flap closure [5,6].

* Corresponding author. Memorial Hospital and Healthcare Center, The Wound Care Center, Jasper, IN.
E-mail address: pvppc@fullnet.com (A. Rader).

0891-8422/08/$ - see front matter © 2008 Elsevier Inc. All rights reserved.
doi:10.1016/j.cpm.2007.10.005

Technique

The authors have used this technique on plantar heel wounds ranging from 2 to 5 cm in diameter. All wounds were initially treated with standard offloading modalities and moist wound-healing principles. In all cases, the cone flap was performed after a fully granular wound free of clinical signs of infection was determined. The patients are required to commit to a 21-day period of non–weight-bearing status on the affected limb. Morbidly obese patients are typically placed into a skilled care facility to assist with non–weight-bearing status.

The surgical technique consists of a rotational fasciocutaneous flap to cover the ulcer. A V-Y fasciocutaneous advancement is then performed to repair the donor site (Figs. 1–4). To avoid edge necrosis of the flaps, the fascia is cut several millimeters larger than the overlying skin. The flap is impossible to advance without incising the plantar fascia circumferentially about the raised flap. Disruption of the vascular supply between the fascia and the skin promotes flap failure. Care is taken to move the fascia, adipose tissue, and skin as a unit while advancement of the flap is performed. All wounds are then closed primarily at the level of the skin only.

Outcomes

Minor wound dehiscence, although uncommon, can occur, and the authors have seen this in their experience. Most of their surgical sites proceeded to uncomplicated healing over a 3-week period. Full weight bearing

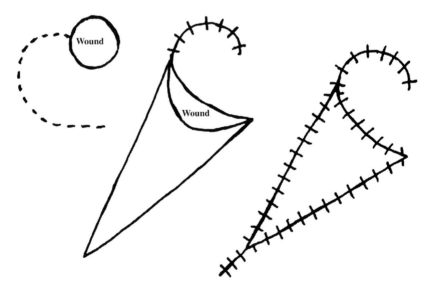

Fig. 1. (*Left*) Defect and pedicle flap design. (*Center*) Rotation of pedicle and V-Y advancement flap design. (*Right*) V-Y flap advancemnt and final closure.

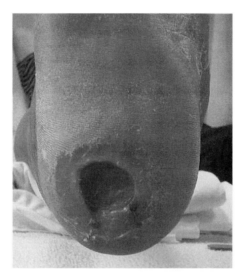

Fig. 2. Plantar heel wound.

at that time has not produced any failures. During the 4-year period the primary author has been performing this flap procedure, no recurrent heel wounds have occurred. These patients all remain enrolled in podiatric care through local wound care centers. Most of the authors' patients have had neuropathic heel wounds, but the authors can recall treating those patients who have had traumatic wounds successfully as well. The patients who have had neuropathic wounds were standardly fitted with appropriate accommodative shoe gear.

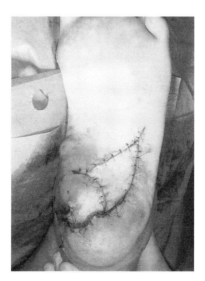

Fig. 3. Intraoperative closure.

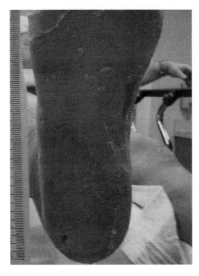

Fig. 4. Postoperative result at 3 weeks.

Discussion

Plantar heel wounds are often difficult to epithelialize in a timely manner. When healing is achieved through secondary intention, the results are often fragile and prone to reulceration. The cone flap provides a surgical option to allow plantar skin coverage for these difficult-to-heal wounds. The fasciocutaneous nature of the flap provides a well-vascularized pedicle for wound coverage. The technique demonstrated requires no specialized training. Understanding the importance of fascia harvesting equal to or slightly larger than the overlying skin is imperative. Following this simple method, a durable primary closure is available to all surgeons who work with chronic foot wounds.

References

[1] Poten B. The fasciocutaneous flap: its use in soft tissue defects of the lower leg. Br J Plast Surg 1981;34:215–20.
[2] Calderon W, Chang N, Mathes S. Comparison of the effects of bacterial inoculation in musculocutaneous and fasciocutaneous flaps. Plast Reconstr Surg 1986;77:785–92.
[3] Wang X, Xia J, Wang D, et al. Vascularity of the fasciocutaneous flap; further delineation of anatomy: blood supply to the skin. Journal of Applied Research in Clinical and Experimental Therapeutics 2001;1(2):48–54.
[4] Schafer K. Das subcutane gefabetasystem (untere extremitant): mikropaparatorische untersuchungen. Gegenbaurs Morphologisches Jahrbuch (Leipzig) 1975;121:492–514 [In German].
[5] Calderon W, Andrades P, Leniz P, et al. The cone flap: a new and versatile fasciocutaneous flap. Plast Reconstr Surg 2004;114(6):1539–42.
[6] Calderon W, Leniz P, Pineros J, et al. The fascio-cutaneous "cone-flap" for treatment of electrical burns. Burns 2007;33(1):S138–9.

ELSEVIER
SAUNDERS

Clin Podiatr Med Surg
25 (2008) 127–133

CLINICS IN
PODIATRIC
MEDICINE AND
SURGERY

The Narrowed Forefoot at 1 Year: An Advanced Approach for Wound Closure After Central Ray Amputations

Nicholas J. Bevilacqua, DPM[a],*,
Lee C. Rogers, DPM[a], Michael P. DellaCorte, DPM[b],
David G. Armstrong, DPM, PhD[c]

[a]*Foot and Ankle Surgery, Amputation Prevention Center, Broadlawns Medical Center,
1801 Hickman Road, Des Moines, IA, USA*
[b]*Caritas Heathcare, Inc., Department of Podiatry, St. Johns Hospital, 90-02 Queens Blvd,
Elmhurst, NY, USA*
[c]*Scholl's Center for Lower Extremity Ambulatory Research at Rosalind Franklin University,
3333 Green Bay Road, North Chicago, IL, USA*

Lower extremity amputation is one of the most feared complications of diabetes. Persons who have diabetes are 15 to 46 times more likely to undergo an amputation than those who do not have diabetes [1–3]. Diabetes is the underlying cause for most lower extremity amputations, and infection is the most common precipitating event [4]. Lower extremity ulcerations act as a portal for infection, insofar as 85% of lower extremity amputations in the United States are preceded by a diabetic foot ulcer [5]. After a lower extremity amputation, 50% of patients undergo contralateral amputation in 2 to 5 years [6]. Postamputation mortality rates range from 13% to 40% after 1 year to as high as 80% after 5 years [7]. A disproportionate share of these adverse outcomes occur in "high-level" or major amputations [8,9], and it has been shown that patients function better with a lower level more distal amputation [10]. Therefore, a prudent surgeon considers function and preserves as much length to the foot as possible.

Treating an infected plantar foot ulcer requires thoroughly evaluating the wound, appropriate antimicrobial therapy, hospitalization, and, often, surgical intervention [4]. Traditional surgical management of plantar forefoot ulcers with underlying osteomyelitis of a lesser metatarsal head

* Corresponding author.
E-mail address: nicholas.bevilacqua@gmail.com (N.J. Bevilacqua).

0891-8422/08/$ - see front matter © 2008 Elsevier Inc. All rights reserved.
doi:10.1016/j.cpm.2007.10.002   *podiatric.theclinics.com*

consisted of partial or complete metatarsal resection, oftentimes resulting in a biomechanically unsound foot accompanied by a cleft wound that is difficult to heal. The resultant unstable foot frequently leads to the development of neuropathic foot ulcerations, resulting in subsequent surgery and, possibly, a high-level amputation. Distal amputations are preferred, and it is imperative the surgeon evaluate the functional outcome and consider the risk for future ulcerations.

The concept of using external fixation for forefoot narrowing was first introduced by Strauss and colleagues [11], which was described for the management of "problem" cleft wounds resulting from resection of a necrotic toe and adjacent metatarsal in 15 patients. These investigators performed adjacent osteotomies, manually compressed the forefoot, and applied a large "cathedral-like configuration" [11]. The wounds were closed primarily and allowed to heal secondarily or covered with a split-thickness skin graft, and 14 of 15 patients received hyperbaric oxygen as an adjunctive therapy. The device remained in place for an average of 27.5 days, followed by 3 weeks of casting. Fourteen patients (87%) resumed ambulation, and the forefoot remained mechanically sound and cosmetically pleasing.

Oznur and Tokgozoglu [12] described a similar technique to that of Strauss and colleagues [11]; they used two Ilizarov external fixation system half-rings instead, however. After third and fourth ray resections, these investigators performed a lateral ray osteotomy and used medial and lateral tensioned olive wires to narrow the forefoot. The wound healed uneventfully, and the external fixator was removed after 8 weeks. The patient remained healed after 4 years of follow-up [12]. Later, Zgonis and colleagues [13] used a similar concept as Oznur and Tokgozoglu [12] but applied a split-thickness skin graft over the remaining soft tissue defect. These investigators removed the external fixation device after maturation of the split-thickness skin graft, which achieved wound closure; however, a cleft foot remained [13].

Bernstein and Guerin [14] presented the use of a light-weight, small, bone-lengthening external fixation device to close central ray defects gradually. These investigators performed weekly manipulation, and the time to closure averaged 30 days.

Methods

The authors retrospectively reviewed the cases of four consecutive patients presenting with plantar forefoot wounds with underlying osteomyelitis to a lesser metatarsal head and treated with central ray resection with forefoot narrowing. Patient characteristics, past medical history, wound classification, time to external fixator removal, and time to complete healing were analyzed. The characteristics of the patients are presented in Table 1. All patients were treated at Saint Vincent Catholic Medical Centers (New York, New York) over the course of 1 year. Institutional Review Board

Table 1
Patient characteristics and results

Patient	Gender	Age (years)	Wound location (submetatarsal number)	Procedure	Time to fixator removal (days)	Follow-up (months)
1	Male	47	3 and 4	Third and fourth ray resection	42	19
2	Male	49	3 and 4	Third ray resection	36	17
3	Male	57	2	Second ray resection	37	16
4	Female	57	3	Third ray resection	30	14
Mean		52.5			36.25	16.5

(IRB) approval was granted by Rosalind Franklin University of Medicine and Science. A typical presentation is shown in Fig. 1.

Surgical technique

Full-thickness incisions are made along the margins of the digit extending proximal and converging dorsal and plantar on the metatarsal shaft. The incision extends further proximally in a plantar direction and incorporates the ulcer. With minimal undermining, the ulcer and digit are removed. The metatarsal is partially resected just distal to the base, the wound is inspected, and all necrotic or infected tissue is debrided [15]. It is important to perform an adequate debridement until the wound edges consist only of normal and healthy tissue [16]. Adjacent osteotomies are not required with

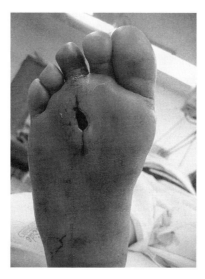

Fig. 1. Initial preoperative presentation.

this technique. The wound is copiously irrigated, and a pulsed lavage system may be used.

An appropriately sized DFS MiniLengthener (Biomet, Parsippany, New Jersey) is chosen. The first and fifth metatarsals are palpated and outlined with a skin scribe for reference. Guided by fluoroscopy, a 3.0-mm, tapered, threaded half-pin is percutaneously driven centrally into the middle to distal one third of the first metatarsal. All pin placements should be perpendicular to the metatarsal and purchase two cortices. Next, a 2.0-mm threaded wire is driven centrally into the distal shaft of the fifth metatarsal. The fixator is loosely secured and serves as a guide for the next half-pin and wire (Fig. 2). Using the proximal clamps, a second 3.0-mm, tapered, threaded half-pin and a 2.0-mm threaded wire are driven into the first and fifth metatarsals, respectively. After verifying the position of all half-pins and wires with fluoroscopy, the external fixator is firmly secured and is placed approximately 2 cm above the dorsum of the foot to allow for postoperative edema [14].

The forefoot is manually compressed until the plantar skin edges appose, and the fixator is closed down to hold the position. The incisions are now primarily closed with nylon suture (Fig. 3). If there is concern regarding residual soft tissue infection, the wound should be left open to drain and the sutures may be tied when deemed appropriate (Fig. 4). Tendo-Achilles lengthening is crucial if it is determined that the Achilles tendon is one of the causative factors that led to the ulceration.

Hospitalized patients are closely monitored; after discharge, patients are seen weekly for dressing changes and pin care, which consists of application of povidone-iodine solution–soaked gauze around the pin sites [13]. The minirail is small and lightweight, allowing the use of a standard surgical shoe. Patients are kept non–weight bearing for approximately 2 weeks (longer if a tendo-Achilles lengthening is performed) and are then transitioned

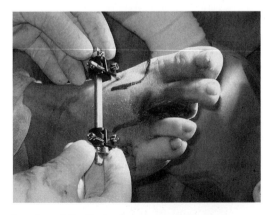

Fig. 2. Intraoperative view of the fixator being secured loosely to serve as a guide for the remaining half-pin and wire.

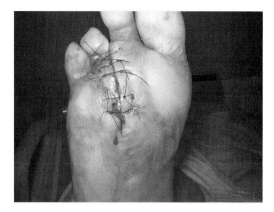

Fig. 3. Sutures may be tied immediately in the operating room or after resolution of infection at bedside.

to partial weight bearing. The external fixator is kept in place until complete healing of the incision and is easily removed in an office or clinic setting (Fig. 5A). The patient is then placed in appropriate footwear.

Results

Over a 19-month period, four patients were treated with the forefoot narrowing technique described previously (see Table 1). The average age of the patients was 53 years (range: 47–57 years). The external fixator was in place for an average of 36 days (range: 30–42 days). Average follow-up was 15

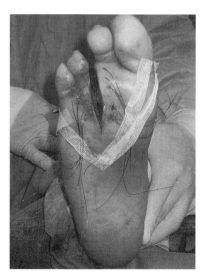

Fig. 4. The wound is left open, and the sutures may be tied when the infection resolves.

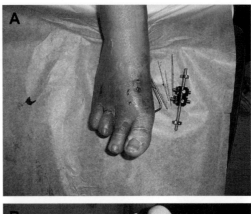

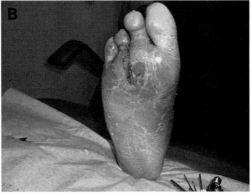

Fig. 5. (*A*) Final appearance of the dorsum of the foot after the fixator has been removed. (*B*) Final appearance of the plantar foot after the fixator has been removed.

months (range: 14–19 months). All four patients healed without additional complications and resumed their previous lifestyle without skin breakdown at follow-up. All four patients were successfully treated, resulting in a flat stable plantar forefoot.

Discussion

Infected diabetic foot ulcers are the most common cause for hospital admission in this population. Diabetic foot problems are a major burden to society and come at great costs to the health care system. Hospital length of stay is longer for diabetic patients who have ulcers when compared with those who do not have ulcers [17]. It is imperative to consider foot structure and assess the risk for future ulcerations in patients undergoing central ray amputations. Oftentimes, after a central ray resection, the resultant foot is mechanically unstable or contains a cleft wound that is difficult to heal [11]. Narrowing the forefoot enables the surgeon to close the plantar defect primarily, thereby eliminating the need for prolonged wound care and lowering the risk for postoperative complications in this high-risk population. This technique allows for immediate wound closure without the need for split-thickness skin grafts and results in a stable plantigrade forefoot and a cosmetically pleasing foot (see Fig. 5). Forefoot narrowing is an effective treatment option for central ray resections, and using this technique may delay the onset of further foot complications.

References

[1] Most RS, Sinnock P. The epidemiology of lower extremity amputations in diabetic individuals. Diabetes Care 1983;6:87–91.

[2] Lavery LA, van Houtum WH, Ashry HR, et al. Diabetes-related lower-extremity amputations disproportionately affect blacks and Mexican Americans. South Med J 1999;92(6): 593–9.

[3] Reiber GE. The epidemiology of diabetic foot problems. Diabet Med 1996;13(Suppl 1): S6–11.

[4] Lavery LA, Armstrong DG, Murdoch DP, et al. Validation of the Infectious Diseases Society of America's diabetic foot infection classification system. Clin Infect Dis 2007;44(4): 562–5.

[5] Pecoraro RE, Reiber GE, Burgess EM. Pathways to diabetic limb amputation: basis for prevention. Diabetes Care 1990;13:513–21.

[6] Larsson J, Agardh CD, Apelqvist J, et al. Long-term prognosis after healed amputation in patients with diabetes. Clin Orthop Relat Res 1998;350:149–58.

[7] Reiber GE. Epidemiology of foot ulcers and amputations in the diabetic foot. In: Bowker JH, Pfeifer MA, editors. The diabetic foot. St. Louis (MO): Mosby; 2001. p. 13–32.

[8] Lavery LA, Van Houtum WH, Harkless LB. In-hospital mortality and disposition of diabetic amputees in the Netherlands. Diabet Med 1996;13:192–7.

[9] Lavery LA, van Houtum WH, Armstrong DG, et al. Mortality following lower extremity amputation in minorities with diabetes mellitus. Diabetes Res Clin Pract 1997;37(1):41–7.

[10] Waters RL, Perry J, Antonelle D, et al. Energy cost of walking of amputees: the influence of level of amputation. J Bone Joint Surg Am 1976;58:42–6.

[11] Strauss MB, Bryant BJ, Hart JD. Forefoot narrowing with external fixation for problem cleft wounds. Foot Ankle Int 2002;23(5):433–9.

[12] Oznur A, Tokgozoglu M. Closure of central defects of the forefoot with external fixation: a case report. J Foot Ankle Surg 2004;43(1):56–9.

[13] Zgonis T, Oznur A, Roukis TS. A novel technique for closing difficult diabetic cleft foot wounds with skin grafting and a ring-type external fixation system. Operative Techniques in Orthopaedics 2006;16:38–43.

[14] Bernstein B, Guerin L. The use of mini external fixation in central forefoot amputations. J Foot Ankle Surg 2005;44(4):307–10.

[15] Attinger CE, Janis JE, Steinberg J, et al. Clinical approach to wounds: debridement and wound bed preparation including the use of dressings and wound-healing adjuvants. Plast Reconstr Surg 2006;117(7 Suppl):72S–109S.

[16] Attinger CE, Bulan EJ. Debridement. The key initial first step in wound healing. Foot Ankle Clin 2001;6(4):627–60.

[17] Reiber GE, Boyko EJ, Smith DG. Lower extremity foot ulcers and amputations in diabetes. In: Harris MI, Cowie C, Stern MP, editors. Diabetes in America. Washington, DC: United Government Printing Office (NIH Publ. 95–1468); 1995. p. 409–28.

ELSEVIER
SAUNDERS

Clin Podiatr Med Surg
25 (2008) 135–137

CLINICS IN
PODIATRIC
MEDICINE AND
SURGERY

Index

Note: Page numbers of article titles are in **boldface** type.

Moving?

Make sure your subscription moves with you!

To notify us of your new address, find your **Clinics Account Number** (located on your mailing label above your name), and contact customer service at:

E-mail: elspcs@elsevier.com

800-654-2452 (subscribers in the U.S. & Canada)
407-345-4000 (subscribers outside of the U.S. & Canada)

Fax number: 407-363-9661

Elsevier Periodicals Customer Service
6277 Sea Harbor Drive
Orlando, FL 32887-4800

*To ensure uninterrupted delivery of your subscription, please notify us at least 4 weeks in advance of move.